Disclaimer Notice:

Please note the information contained within this document is for educational and entertainment purposes only. All effort has been executed to present accurate, up to date, reliable, complete information. No warranties of any kind are declared or implied. Readers acknowledge that the author is not engaged in the rendering of legal, financial, medical, or professional advice. The content within this book has been derived from various sources. Please consult a licensed professional before attempting any techniques outlined in this book.

By reading this document, the reader agrees that under no circumstances is the author responsible for any losses, direct or indirect, that are incurred as a result of the use of the information contained within this document, including, but not limited to, errors, omissions, or inaccuracies.

CONTENTS

What is the Mediterranean diet? Main guidelines, foods to eat and what to avoid

If you are searching for a healthy way to lose the weight and to maintain an optimal health, then this is the best diet for you. It's the Mediterranean diet, a very popular and unique one.

The Mediterranean diet is mainly based on the foods people from countries like Italy and Greece used to eat back in the '60s. Researches in the field proved that these were extremely healthy and that they had a very low risk of many illnesses. Besides the fact that the Mediterranean diet can help you lose the extra weight, it can also prevent the appearance of heart related illnesses, strokes and even diabetes.

This healthy lifestyle is based on consuming easy to find products that are full of important nutrients, vitamins and antioxidants. All these contribute to a healthy body and appearance.

One of the best things about this exceptional diet is that it's not an expensive one. It's actually a budget friendly one that uses accessible ingredients everyone can manage.

The Mediterranean lifestyle encourages physical exercise and enjoying the meals you make with friends and family.

The diet has few limitations and it allows a lot of experimentation with ingredients and flavors.

Now that you are familiarized with this diet and with its main principles, it's time you knew what you can and can not eat.

Basically, you can eat all kinds of vegetables, nuts, seeds, fruits, whole, grains, legumes, herbs, fish, seafood and healthy foods.

You should consume in moderation eggs, poultry, pork, cheese, sour cream, heavy cream and yogurt and you should almost never eat beef.

You should never eat processed meat, sweetened beverages, refined oil or processed foods.

Always avoid sodas, candies, ice cream, white bread, refined wheat, margarines and other trans fats, canola oil, soybean oil, hot dogs and anything labeled low-fat or diet.

These are the main products you can and can not consume during the Mediterranean diet, but we thought you could use more specific guidelines as well.

Therefore, here are the ingredients you should base your Mediterranean diet meals on!

When it comes to veggies, there are a lot of options. You can eat tomatoes, eggplants, kale, broccoli, spinach, cauliflower, cucumbers, avocados, carrots, Brussels sprouts, parsnips, turnips, artichokes, endives, fennels, etc.

As far as fruits are concerned, feel free to eat as many apples, oranges, pears, bananas, grapes, strawberries, blueberries, blackberries, melons, peaches, apricots, figs or dates as you like.

Also, you can consume walnuts, almonds, hazelnuts, pumpkin seeds, sunflower seeds, cashews, macadamia nuts, chia seeds, hemp seeds, etc.

Make sure your meals also contain peas, all kind of beans, chickpeas, peanuts, lentils.

Don't forget you can make delicious meals using yams, sweet potatoes and regular potatoes.

Whole oats, rice, rye, barley, corn, whole wheat, quinoa and bulgur are also a must if following the Mediterranean diet.

Last but not least, consume shrimp, clams, crab, mussels, sardines, salmon, tuna, trout, mackerel or oysters.

Consume chicken, duck, turkey, pork, lamb, eggs, cheese, yogurt and Greek yogurt as well.

Season your foods with salt, pepper, garlic, mint, basil, sage, rosemary, nutmeg, cinnamon, saffron, turmeric, cumin, peppercorns, fennel seeds, etc.

Use healthy oils like avocado or olive oil ones.

If you decide that the Mediterranean lifestyle suits you, make sure you drink enough water during the day. You can also drink moderate amounts of wine (mostly red wine), coffee and tea. Just make sure that you don't consume sweetened beverages and fruits juices that contain a lot of sugar.

Snacks should be included in a Mediterranean diet plan. Some great snack ideas would be a serving of nuts, fruits like plums and grapes, dried fruits like apricots, hummus with veggie sticks or mashed avocado on whole wheat toast.

Now that you know what you can eat on a Mediterranean diet, it's time to find out which foods you have to avoid.

First of all, red meat shouldn't be an option on a Mediterranean diet. You will have to avoid beef as much as possible. Also, try to limit the consumption of processed meat like sausages or salami.

Avoid added sugars if you want to stick to your healthy diet. This means you have to stay away from candy, baked goods and sweetened drinks like soda.

Use honey, stevia and even cinnamon to sweeten your desserts, tea and coffee.

Make sure you don't use white flour or refined grains like white rice. These have a lower nutritional value and they don't contain the fibers you need. You can replace them with brown rice, whole wheat grains and almond flour.

Last but not least, try to replace the butter with olive oil. This will suit the Mediterranean diet better.

As you can see, this diet doesn't have as many restrictions as you might think but these guidelines should be followed in order to enjoy the health benefits and weight loss.

The Mediterranean diet limits the meat consumption and is based on eating a lot of veggies and fruits. Therefore, this diet is suitable for vegans and vegetarians as well.

So, if you are a vegan who wants to start a Mediterranean diet you can consume nuts, seeds, tofu and even beans. It's actually pretty easy to follow this diet if you are a vegan. All you have to do is to focus on eating certain foods. First of all, you can consume a lot of beans because they contain healthy proteins and fibers. They prevent the appearance of heart related issues and they are vital for such a diet. Use them to make salads, sautés, soups and stews.

You can also consume tofu as a meat replacement. Add small servings of tofu to you meals a few times per week. Nuts and seeds are a great option if you are a vegan on a Mediterranean diet. They provide the omega-3 you need in order to stay healthy. include flaxseeds, walnuts, hemp seeds and chia seeds to your diet.

Also, add fibers and whole grains to you diet in order to feel full and satisfied longer. Eat more quinoa, whole wheat pasta and whole wheat bread.

Veggies are extremely important if you are a vegan following such a diet. Consume as many veggies as you like because they contain all the vitamins a vegan needs.

If you are a vegan you can eat as many fruits as you like. These are not just healthy but they can also satisfy your sweet tooth. Fruits like berries, oranges, grapefruits or raspberries contain a lot of vitamins and antioxidants and they should be included in your diet.

Last but not least, try to see this diet as a healthy lifestyle. Embrace it and make it your own. We guarantee it will soon show its amazing benefits.

The Mediterranean diet can change your life, it can definitely improve your healthy, your appearance and your metabolism. You simply must make sure you consume the foods allowed and that you avoid anything that can interfere with the success of this diet.

That's a simple formula of success and anyone can follow such a diet. It's not a complex one and it will make you feel so much different in no time.

If you made the decision to opt for the Mediterranean diet, you might need to know something more. There are some tips and tricks that will help you stay on your diet and enjoy it. Also, you might want to know what to include in your shopping list and what to eat when you go out with friends and you are on the Mediterranean diet.

Check this out!

Tips& Tricks To Help You Follow The Mediterranean Diet

Here are some useful tips and tricks to help you follow the Mediterranean diet. They will really come in hand once you decide that Mediterranean lifestyle suit you.

If you are on such a diet and you want to enjoy a night out at a restaurant with your friends, here's what you can do. First of all, opt for fish and seafood as a main dish. You can't go wrong with this. Also, ask the personnel to use olive oil in your foods and only consume whole grain bread.

We guarantee that you can't go wrong with this. You will enjoy a lovely night out and you will still stick to your diet.

Another great idea to keep in mind when you are on such a diet is to make a great shopping list. It will help you buy the right ingredients. Choose organic products if you can but only if they suit your budget.

Your shopping list must include:

- Veggies like kale, garlic, spinach, arugula, onions, carrots
- Fruits like grapes, oranges, apples and bananas
- Berries like blueberries, strawberries, raspberries
- Frozen veggies
- Grains like whole-grain pasta, whole-grain breads
- Legumes like beans, lentils, chickpeas
- Nuts like walnuts, cashews, almonds
- Seeds like pumpkin seeds and sunflower seeds
- Condiments like turmeric, cinnamon, salt, pepper
- Shrimp and shellfish
- Fish like mackerel, trout, tuna, salmon and sardines
- Cheese
- Yogurt and Greek yogurt
- Potatoes and sweet potatoes
- Chicken
- Eggs
- Olives
- Olive oil and avocado oil

If you buy healthy and adequate ingredients, you will most certainly eat the right foods and you will definitely stay on your diet.

Now that you also know what to buy if you are on a Mediterranean diet it's time to discover some simple tricks and tips that will make things easier.

1. Keeping in mind that you can not eat red meat, you can replace it with salmon. It will satisfy your cravings but it will allow you to stay on your diet.
2. Make sure you always have olive oil at hand. You have to forget about using butter if you are on the Mediterranean diet but you can replace it with the extra virgin olive oil.
3. Give up consuming sodas and replace them with some red wine. Cut out the sweet drinks from your diet and try one glass of red wine instead.
4. If you are on a Mediterranean diet, you should try to consume more avocados. Avocados contain healthy fats and can be used in so many different ways.
5. You know that you can't eat too much food on a Mediterranean diet but here's something you can try if you can't stay away from meat for too long. Try to avoid eating meat at least one day per week (Monday, for example).
6. Make sure you have all your favorite spices at hand. Stock up your pantry with spices and condiments like paprika, cayenne, chili flakes, turmeric or saffron that will help you get those Mediterranean flavors you crave for.
7. Replace white rice with brown rice. The Mediterranean diet allows you to continue to eat rice but make sure you replace the white rice with brown one. Consume whole grains like buckwheat, corn and quinoa.
8. Your snacks should mainly contain fruits. Consume more citrus, melons, berries or grapes. You can also try seeds as a Mediterranean diet snack but fruits would be a better option.
9. Legumes and beans must be an option. One of the best parts of the Mediterranean diet is exactly this: the consumption of more legumes and beans.
10. Exercise a lot and drink plenty of water. This is a main principle to follow if you are on a Mediterranean diet. It will help you look better and feel amazing. That's a fact!
11. Last but not least, a good trick that will help you really embrace the Mediterranean lifestyle is to take your time and enjoy your meals. This is a great thing to keep in mind. This way you will be able to savor your meals.

We can assure you that if you follow our tips and tricks, you will manage to follow this diet in a fun and easy way. You should see the Mediterranean diet as a new, healthy lifestyle that will change your looks and improve your health. You should enjoy your meals, you should play with ingredients, flavors and textures. This way you will get real Mediterranean culinary feasts.

In order to help you with this, we managed to gather 550 of the best and most delicious Mediterranean diet meals you can ever have. Try them all and be amazed! Have fun cooking the Mediterranean way and enjoy your meals!

Breakfast Recipes

Eggs with Zucchini Noodles

Preparation time: 10 minutes
Cooking time: 11 minutes
Servings: 2
Ingredients:

- 2 tablespoons extra-virgin olive oil
- 3 zucchinis, cut with a spiralizer
- 4 eggs
- Salt and black pepper to the taste
- A pinch of red pepper flakes
- Cooking spray
- 1 tablespoon basil, chopped

Directions:
1. In a bowl, combine the zucchini noodles with salt, pepper and the olive oil and toss well.
2. Grease a baking sheet with cooking spray and divide the zucchini noodles into 4 nests on it.
3. Crack an egg on top of each nest, sprinkle salt, pepper and the pepper flakes on top and bake at 350 degrees F for 11 minutes.
4. Divide the mix between plates, sprinkle the basil on top and serve.
Nutrition: calories 296, fat 23.6, fiber 3.3, carbs 10.6, protein 14.7

Banana Oats

Preparation time: 10 minutes
Cooking time: 0 minutes
Servings: 2
Ingredients:

- 1 banana, peeled and sliced
- ¾ cup almond milk
- ½ cup cold brewed coffee
- 2 dates, pitted
- 2 tablespoons cocoa powder
- 1 cup rolled oats
- 1 and ½ tablespoons chia seeds

Directions:
1. In a blender, combine the banana with the milk and the rest of the ingredients, pulse, divide into bowls and serve for breakfast.
Nutrition: calories 451, fat 25.1, fiber 9.9, carbs 55.4, protein 9.3

Slow-cooked Peppers Frittata

Preparation time: 10 minutes
Cooking time: 3 hours
Servings: 6
Ingredients:

- ½ cup almond milk
- 8 eggs, whisked
- Salt and black pepper to the taste
- 1 teaspoon oregano, dried
- 1 and ½ cups roasted peppers, chopped
- ½ cup red onion, chopped
- 4 cups baby arugula

- 1 cup goat cheese, crumbled
- Cooking spray

Directions:
1. In a bowl, combine the eggs with salt, pepper and the oregano and whisk.
2. Grease your slow cooker with the cooking spray, arrange the peppers and the remaining ingredients inside and pour the eggs mixture over them.
3. Put the lid on and cook on Low for 3 hours.
4. Divide the frittata between plates and serve.
Nutrition: calories 259, fat 20.2, fiber 1, carbs 4.4, protein 16.3

Veggie Bowls

Preparation time: 10 minutes
Cooking time: 5 minutes
Servings: 4
Ingredients:

- 1 tablespoon olive oil
- 1 pound asparagus, trimmed and roughly chopped
- 3 cups kale, shredded
- 3 cups Brussels sprouts, shredded
- ½ cup hummus
- 1 avocado, peeled, pitted and sliced
- 4 eggs, soft boiled, peeled and sliced

For the dressing:

- 2 tablespoons lemon juice
- 1 garlic clove, minced
- 2 teaspoons Dijon mustard
- 2 tablespoons olive oil
- Salt and black pepper to the taste

Directions:
1. Heat up a pan with 2 tablespoons oil over medium-high heat, add the asparagus and sauté for 5 minutes stirring often.
2. In a bowl, combine the other 2 tablespoons oil with the lemon juice, garlic, mustard, salt and pepper and whisk well.
3. In a salad bowl, combine the asparagus with the kale, sprouts, hummus, avocado and the eggs and toss gently.
4. Add the dressing, toss and serve for breakfast.
Nutrition: calories 323, fat 21, fiber 10.9, carbs 24.8

Avocado and Apple Smoothie

Preparation time: 5 minutes
Cooking time: 0 minutes
Servings: 2
Ingredients:

- 3 cups spinach
- 1 green apple, cored and chopped
- 1 avocado, peeled, pitted and chopped
- 3 tablespoons chia seeds
- 1 teaspoon honey
- 1 banana, frozen and peeled
- 2 cups coconut water

Directions:

1. In your blender, combine the spinach with the apple and the rest of the ingredients, pulse, divide into glasses and serve.
Nutrition: calories 168, fat 10.1, fiber 6, carbs 21, protein 2.1

Avocado Toast

Preparation time: 10 minutes
Cooking time: 0 minutes
Servings: 2
Ingredients:
- 1 tablespoon goat cheese, crumbled
- 1 avocado, peeled, pitted and mashed
- A pinch of salt and black pepper
- 2 whole wheat bread slices, toasted
- ½ teaspoon lime juice
- 1 persimmon, thinly sliced
- 1 fennel bulb, thinly sliced
- 2 teaspoons honey
- 2 tablespoons pomegranate seeds

Directions:
1. In a bowl, combine the avocado flesh with salt, pepper, lime juice and the cheese and whisk.
2. Spread this onto toasted bread slices, top each slice with the remaining ingredients and serve for breakfast.
Nutrition: calories 348, fat 20.8, fiber 12.3, carbs 38.7, protein 7.1

Mini Frittatas

Preparation time: 5 minutes
Cooking time: 15 minutes
Servings: 12
Ingredients:
- 1 yellow onion, chopped
- 1 cup parmesan, grated
- 1 yellow bell pepper, chopped
- 1 red bell pepper, chopped
- 1 zucchini, chopped
- Salt and black pepper to the taste
- 8 eggs, whisked
- A drizzle of olive oil
- 2 tablespoons chives, chopped

Directions:
1. Heat up a pan with the oil over medium-high heat, add the onion, the zucchini and the rest of the ingredients except the eggs and chives and sauté for 5 minutes stirring often.
2. Divide this mix on the bottom of a muffin pan, pour the eggs mixture on top, sprinkle salt, pepper and the chives and bake at 350 degrees F for 10 minutes.
3. Serve the mini frittatas for breakfast right away.
Nutrition: calories 55, fat 3, fiber 0.7, carbs 3.2, protein 4.2

Berry Oats

Preparation time: 5 minutes
Cooking time: 0 minutes
Servings: 2

Ingredients:
- ½ cup rolled oats
- 1 cup almond milk
- ¼ cup chia seeds
- A pinch of cinnamon powder
- 2 teaspoons honey
- 1 cup berries, pureed
- 1 tablespoon yogurt

Directions:
1. In a bowl, combine the oats with the milk and the rest of the ingredients except the yogurt, toss, divide into bowls, top with the yogurt and serve cold for breakfast.
Nutrition: calories 420, fat 30.3, fiber 7.2, carbs 35.3, protein 6.4

Sun-dried Tomatoes Oatmeal

Preparation time: 10 minutes
Cooking time: 25 minutes
Servings: 4
Ingredients:
- 3 cups water
- 1 cup almond milk
- 1 tablespoon olive oil
- 1 cup steel-cut oats
- ¼ cup sun-dried tomatoes, chopped
- A pinch of red pepper flakes

Directions:
1. In a pan, mix the water with the milk, bring to a boil over medium heat.
2. Meanwhile, heat up a pan with the oil over medium-high heat, add the oats, cook them for about 2 minutes and transfer m to the pan with the milk.
3. Stir the oats, add the tomatoes and simmer over medium heat for 23 minutes.
4. Divide the mix into bowls, sprinkle the red pepper flakes on top and serve for breakfast.
Nutrition: calories 170, fat 17.8, fiber 1.5, carbs 3.8, protein 1.5

Quinoa Muffins

Preparation time: 10 minutes
Cooking time: 30 minutes
Servings: 12
Ingredients:
- 1 cup quinoa, cooked
- 6 eggs, whisked
- Salt and black pepper to the taste
- 1 cup Swiss cheese, grated
- 1 small yellow onion, chopped
- 1 cup white mushrooms, sliced
- ½ cup sun-dried tomatoes, chopped

Directions:
1. In a bowl, combine the eggs with salt, pepper and the rest of the ingredients and whisk well.
2. Divide this into a silicone muffin pan, bake at 350 degrees F for 30 minutes and serve for breakfast.
Nutrition: calories 123, fat 5.6, fiber 1.3, carbs 10.8, protein 7.5

Quinoa and Eggs Pan

Preparation time: 10 minutes
Cooking time: 23 minutes
Servings: 4
Ingredients:
- 4 bacon slices, cooked and crumbled
- A drizzle of olive oil
- 1 small red onion, chopped
- 1 red bell pepper, chopped
- 1 sweet potato, grated
- 1 green bell pepper, chopped
- 2 garlic cloves, minced
- 1 cup white mushrooms, sliced
- ½ cup quinoa
- 1 cup chicken stock
- 4 eggs, fried
- Salt and black pepper to the taste

Directions:
1. Heat up a pan with the oil over medium-low heat, add the onion, garlic, bell peppers, sweet potato and the mushrooms, toss and sauté for 5 minutes.
2. Add the quinoa, toss and cook for 1 more minute.
3. Add the stock, salt and pepper, stir and cook for 15 minutes.
4. Divide the mix between plates, top each serving with a fried egg, sprinkle some salt, pepper and crumbled bacon and serve for breakfast.
Nutrition: calories 304, fat 14, fiber 3.8, carbs 27.5, protein 17.8

Stuffed Tomatoes

Preparation time: 10 minutes
Cooking time: 15 minutes
Servings: 4
Ingredients:
- 2 tablespoons olive oil
- 8 tomatoes, insides scooped
- ¼ cup almond milk
- 8 eggs
- ¼ cup parmesan, grated
- Salt and black pepper to the taste
- 4 tablespoons rosemary, chopped

Directions:
1. Grease a pan with the oil and arrange the tomatoes inside.
2. Crack an egg in each tomato, divide the milk and the rest of the ingredients, introduce the pan in the oven and bake at 375 degrees F for 15 minutes.
3. Serve for breakfast right away.
Nutrition: calories 276, fat 20.3, fiber 4.7, carbs 13.2, protein 13.7

Scrambled Eggs

Preparation time: 10 minutes
Cooking time: 10 minutes
Servings: 2
Ingredients:
- 1 yellow bell pepper, chopped
- 8 cherry tomatoes, cubed
- 2 spring onions, chopped
- 1 tablespoon olive oil
- 1 tablespoon capers, drained
- 2 tablespoons black olives, pitted and sliced
- 4 eggs
- A pinch of salt and black pepper
- ¼ teaspoon oregano, dried
- 1 tablespoon parsley, chopped

Directions:
1. Heat up a pan with the oil over medium-high heat, add the bell pepper and spring onions and sauté for 3 minutes.
2. Add the tomatoes, capers and the olives and sauté for 2 minutes more.
3. Crack the eggs into the pan, add salt, pepper and the oregano and scramble for 5 minutes more.
4. Divide the scramble between plates, sprinkle the parsley on top and serve.
Nutrition: calories 249, fat 17, fiber 3.2, carbs 13.3, protein 13.5

Watermelon "Pizza"

Preparation time: 10 minutes
Cooking time: 0 minutes
Servings: 4
Ingredients:
- 1 watermelon slice cut 1-inch thick and then from the center cut into 4 wedges resembling pizza slices
- 6 kalamata olives, pitted and sliced
- 1 ounce feta cheese, crumbled
- ½ tablespoon balsamic vinegar
- 1 teaspoon mint, chopped

Directions:
1. Arrange the watermelon "pizza" on a plate, sprinkle the olives and the rest of the ingredients on each slice and serve right away for breakfast.
Nutrition: calories 90, fat 3, fiber 1, carbs 14, protein 2

Ham Muffins

Preparation time: 10 minutes
Cooking time: 15 minutes
Servings: 6
Ingredients:
- 9 ham slices
- 5 eggs, whisked
- 1/3 cup spinach, chopped
- ¼ cup feta cheese, crumbled
- ½ cup roasted red peppers, chopped
- A pinch of salt and black pepper
- 1 and ½ tablespoons basil pesto
- Cooking spray

Directions:
1. Grease a muffin tin with cooking spray and line each muffin mould with 1 and ½ ham slices.
2. Divide the peppers and the rest of the ingredients except the eggs, pesto, salt and pepper into the ham cups.

3. In a bowl, mix the eggs with the pesto, salt and pepper, whisk and pour over the peppers mix.
4. Bake the muffins in the oven at 400 degrees F for 15 minutes and serve for breakfast.
Nutrition: calories 109, fat 6.7, fiber 1.8, carbs 1.8, protein 9.3

Avocado Chickpea Pizza

Preparation time: 20 minutes
Cooking time: 20 minutes
Servings: 2
Ingredients:
- 1 and ¼ cups chickpea flour
- A pinch of salt and black pepper
- 1 and ¼ cups water
- 2 tablespoons olive oil
- 1 teaspoon onion powder
- 1 teaspoon garlic, minced
- 1 tomato, sliced
- 1 avocado, peeled, pitted and sliced
- 2 ounces gouda, sliced
- ¼ cup tomato sauce
- 2 tablespoons green onions, chopped

Directions:
1. In a bowl, mix the chickpea flour with salt, pepper, water, the oil, onion powder and the garlic, stir well until you obtain a dough, knead a bit, put in a bowl, cover and leave aside for 20 minutes.
2. Transfer the dough to a working surface, shape a bit circle, transfer it to a baking sheet lined with parchment paper and bake at 425 degrees F for 10 minutes.
3. Spread the tomato sauce over the pizza, also spread the rest of the ingredients and bake at 400 degrees F for 10 minutes more.
4. Cut and serve for breakfast.
Nutrition: calories 416, fat 24.5, fiber 9.6, carbs 36.6, protein 15.4

Banana and Quinoa Casserole

Preparation time: 10 minutes
Cooking time: 1 hour and 20 minutes
Servings: 8
Ingredients:
- 3 cups bananas, peeled and mashed
- ¼ cup pure maple syrup
- ¼ cup molasses
- 1 tablespoon cinnamon powder
- 2 teaspoons vanilla extract
- 1 teaspoon cloves, ground
- 1 teaspoon ginger, ground
- ½ teaspoon allspice, ground
- 1 cup quinoa
- ¼ cup almonds, chopped
- 2 and ½ cups almond milk

Directions:
1. In a baking dish, combine the bananas with the maple syrup, molasses and the rest of the ingredients, toss and bake at 350 degrees F for 1 hour and 20 minutes.

2. Divide the mix between plates and serve for breakfast.
Nutrition: calories 213, fat 4.1, fiber 4, carbs 41, protein 4.5

Spiced Chickpeas Bowls

Preparation time: 10 minutes
Cooking time: 30 minutes
Servings: 4
Ingredients:
- 15 ounces canned chickpeas, drained and rinsed
- ¼ teaspoon cardamom, ground
- ½ teaspoon cinnamon powder
- 1 and ½ teaspoons turmeric powder
- 1 teaspoon coriander, ground
- 1 tablespoon olive oil
- A pinch of salt and black pepper
- ¾ cup Greek yogurt
- ½ cup green olives, pitted and halved
- ½ cup cherry tomatoes, halved
- 1 cucumber, sliced

Directions:
1. Spread the chickpeas on a lined baking sheet, add the cardamom, cinnamon, turmeric, coriander, the oil, salt and pepper, toss and bake at 375 degrees F for 30 minutes.
2. In a bowl, combine the roasted chickpeas with the rest of the ingredients, toss and serve for breakfast.
Nutrition: calories 519, fat 34.5, fiber 13.3, carbs 49.8, protein 12

Avocado Spread

Preparation time: 5 minutes
Cooking time: 0 minutes
Servings: 8
Ingredients:
- 2 avocados, peeled, pitted and roughly chopped
- 1 tablespoon sun-dried tomatoes, chopped
- 2 tablespoons lemon juice
- 3 tablespoons cherry tomatoes, chopped
- ¼ cup red onion, chopped
- 1 teaspoon oregano, dried
- 2 tablespoons parsley, chopped
- 4 kalamata olives, pitted and chopped
- A pinch of salt and black pepper

Directions:
1. Put the avocados in a bowl and mash with a fork.
2. Add the rest of the ingredients, stir to combine and serve as a morning spread.
Nutrition: calories 110, fat 10, fiber 3.8, carbs 5.7, protein 1.2

Cheesy Yogurt

Preparation time: 4 hours and 5 minutes
Cooking time: 0 minutes
Servings: 4
Ingredients:

- 1 cup Greek yogurt
- 1 tablespoon honey
- ½ cup feta cheese, crumbled

Directions:
1. In a blender, combine the yogurt with the honey and the cheese and pulse well.
2. Divide into bowls and freeze for 4 hours before serving for breakfast.

Nutrition: calories 161, fat 10, fiber 0, carbs 11.8, protein 6.6

Baked Omelet Mix

Preparation time: 10 minutes
Cooking time: 45 minutes
Servings: 12
Ingredients:
- 12 eggs, whisked
- 8 ounces spinach, chopped
- 2 cups almond milk
- 12 ounces canned artichokes, chopped
- 2 garlic cloves, minced
- 5 ounces feta cheese, crumbled
- 1 tablespoon dill, chopped
- 1 teaspoon oregano, dried
- 1 teaspoon lemon pepper
- A pinch of salt
- 4 teaspoons olive oil

Directions:
1. Heat up a pan with the oil over medium-high heat, add the garlic and the spinach and sauté for 3 minutes.
2. In a baking dish, combine the eggs with the artichokes and the rest of the ingredients.
3. Add the spinach mix as well, toss a bit, bake the mix at 375 degrees F for 40 minutes, divide between plates and serve for breakfast.

Nutrition: calories 186, fat 13, fiber 1, carbs 5, protein 10

Stuffed Sweet Potato

Preparation time: 10 minutes
Cooking time: 40 minutes
Servings: 8
Ingredients:
- 8 sweet potatoes, pierced with a fork
- 14 ounces canned chickpeas, drained and rinsed
- 1 small red bell pepper, chopped
- 1 tablespoon lemon zest, grated
- 2 tablespoons lemon juice
- 3 tablespoons olive oil
- 1 teaspoon garlic, minced
- 1 tablespoon oregano, chopped
- 2 tablespoons parsley, chopped
- A pinch of salt and black pepper
- 1 avocado, peeled, pitted and mashed
- ¼ cup water
- ¼ cup tahini paste

Directions:

1. Arrange the potatoes on a baking sheet lined with parchment paper, bake them at 400 degrees F for 40 minutes, cool them down and cut a slit down the middle in each.
2. In a bowl, combine the chickpeas with the bell pepper, lemon zest, half of the lemon juice, half of the oil, half of the garlic, oregano, half of the parsley, salt and pepper, toss and stuff the potatoes with this mix.
3. In another bowl, mix the avocado with the water, tahini, the rest of the lemon juice, oil, garlic and parsley, whisk well and spread over the potatoes.
4. Serve cold for breakfast.

Nutrition: calories 308, fat 2, fiber 8, carbs 38, protein 7

Cauliflower Fritters

Preparation time: 10 minutes
Cooking time: 50 minutes
Servings: 4
Ingredients:
- 30 ounces canned chickpeas, drained and rinsed
- 2 and ½ tablespoons olive oil
- 1 small yellow onion, chopped
- 2 cups cauliflower florets chopped
- 2 tablespoons garlic, minced
- A pinch of salt and black pepper

Directions:
1. Spread half of the chickpeas on a baking sheet lined with parchment pepper, add 1 tablespoon oil, season with salt and pepper, toss and bake at 400 degrees F for 30 minutes.
2. Transfer the chickpeas to a food processor, pulse well and put the mix into a bowl.
3. Heat up a pan with the ½ tablespoon oil over medium-high heat, add the garlic and the onion and sauté for 3 minutes.
4. Add the cauliflower, cook for 6 minutes more, transfer this to a blender, add the rest of the chickpeas, pulse, pour over the crispy chickpeas mix from the bowl, stir and shape medium fritters out of this mix.
5. Heat up a pan with the rest of the oil over medium-high heat, add the fritters, cook them for 3 minutes on each side and serve for breakfast.

Nutrition: calories 333, fat 12.6, fiber 12.8, carbs 44.7, protein 13.6

Tuna Salad

Preparation time: 10 minutes
Cooking time: 0 minutes
Servings: 2
Ingredients:
- 12 ounces canned tuna in water, drained and flaked
- ¼ cup roasted red peppers, chopped
- 2 tablespoons capers, drained
- 8 kalamata olives, pitted and sliced
- 2 tablespoons olive oil
- 1 tablespoon parsley, chopped
- 1 tablespoon lemon juice

- A pinch of salt and black pepper

Directions:
1. In a bowl, combine the tuna with roasted peppers and the rest of the ingredients, toss, divide between plates and serve for breakfast.

Nutrition: calories 250, fat 17.3, fiber 0.8, carbs 2.7, protein 10.1

Veggie Quiche

Preparation time: 6 minutes
Cooking time: 55 minutes
Servings: 8
Ingredients:
- ½ cup sun-dried tomatoes, chopped
- 1 prepared pie crust
- 2 tablespoons avocado oil
- 1 yellow onion, chopped
- 2 garlic cloves, minced
- 2 cups spinach, chopped
- 1 red bell pepper, chopped
- ¼ cup kalamata olives, pitted and sliced
- 1 teaspoon parsley flakes
- 1 teaspoon oregano, dried
- 1/3 cup feta cheese, crumbled
- 4 eggs, whisked
- 1 and ½ cups almond milk
- 1 cup cheddar cheese, shredded
- Salt and black pepper to the taste

Directions:
1. Heat up a pan with the oil over medium-high heat, add the garlic and onion and sauté for 3 minutes.
2. Add the bell pepper and sauté for 3 minutes more.
3. Add the olives, parsley, spinach, oregano, salt and pepper and cook everything for 5 minutes.
4. Add tomatoes and the cheese, toss and take off the heat.
5. Arrange the pie crust in a pie plate, pour the spinach and tomatoes mix inside and spread.
6. In a bowl, mix the eggs with salt, pepper, the milk and half of the cheese, whisk and pour over the mixture in the pie crust.
7. Sprinkle the remaining cheese on top and bake at 375 degrees F for 40 minutes.
8. Cool the quiche down, slice and serve for breakfast.

Nutrition: calories 211, fat 14.4, fiber 1.4, carbs 12.5, protein 8.6

Potato Hash

Preparation time: 10 minutes
Cooking time: 15 minutes
Servings: 4
Ingredients:
- A drizzle of olive oil
- 2 gold potatoes, cubed
- 2 garlic cloves, minced
- 1 yellow onion, chopped
- 1 cup canned chickpeas, drained

- Salt and black pepper to the taste
- 1 and ½ teaspoon allspice, ground
- 1 pound baby asparagus, trimmed and chopped
- 1 teaspoon sweet paprika
- 1 teaspoon oregano, dried
- 1 teaspoon coriander, ground
- 2 tomatoes, cubed
- 1 cup parsley, chopped
- ½ cup feta cheese, crumbled

Directions:
1. Heat up a pan with a drizzle of oil over medium-high heat, add the potatoes, onion, garlic, salt and pepper and cook for 7 minutes.
2. Add the rest of the ingredients except the tomatoes, parsley and the cheese, toss, cook for 7 more minutes and transfer to a bowl.
3. Add the remaining ingredients, toss and serve for breakfast.

Nutrition: calories 535, fat 20.8, fiber 6.6, carbs 34.5, protein 26.6

Leeks and Eggs Muffins

Preparation time: 10 minutes
Cooking time: 20 minutes
Servings: 2
Ingredients:
- 3 eggs, whisked
- ¼ cup baby spinach
- 2 tablespoons leeks, chopped
- 4 tablespoons parmesan, grated
- 2 tablespoons almond milk
- Cooking spray
- 1 small red bell pepper, chopped
- Salt and black pepper to the taste
- 1 tomato, cubed
- 2 tablespoons cheddar cheese, grated

Directions:
1. In a bowl, combine the eggs with the milk, salt, pepper and the rest of the ingredients except the cooking spray and whisk well.
2. Grease a muffin tin with the cooking spray and divide the eggs mixture in each muffin mould.
3. Bake at 380 degrees F for 20 minutes and serve them for breakfast.

Nutrition: calories 308, fat 19.4, fiber 1.7, carbs 8.7, protein 24.4

Artichokes and Cheese Omelet

Preparation time: 10 minutes
Cooking time: 8 minutes
Servings: 1
Ingredients:
- 1 teaspoon avocado oil
- 1 tablespoon almond milk
- 2 eggs, whisked
- A pinch of salt and black pepper
- 2 tablespoons tomato, cubed
- 2 tablespoons kalamata olives, pitted and sliced
- 1 artichoke heart, chopped
- 1 tablespoon tomato sauce

- 1 tablespoon feta cheese, crumbled

Directions:

1.   In a bowl, combine the eggs with the milk, salt, pepper and the rest of the ingredients except the avocado oil and whisk well.

2.   Heat up a pan with the avocado oil over medium-high heat, add the omelet mix, spread into the pan, cook for 4 minutes, flip, cook for 4 minutes more, transfer to a plate and serve.

Nutrition: calories 303, fat 17.7, fiber 9.9, carbs 21.9, protein 18.2

Quinoa and Eggs Salad

Preparation time: 5 minutes
Cooking time: 0 minutes
Servings: 4
Ingredients:

- 4 eggs, soft boiled, peeled and cut into wedges
- 2 cups baby arugula
- 2 cups cherry tomatoes, halved
- 1 cucumber, sliced
- 1 cup quinoa, cooked
- 1 cup almonds, chopped
- 1 avocado, peeled, pitted and sliced
- 1 tablespoon olive oil
- ½ cup mixed dill and mint, chopped
- A pinch of salt and black pepper
- Juice of 1 lemon

Directions:

1.   In a large salad bowl, combine the eggs with the arugula and the rest of the ingredients, toss, divide between plates and serve for breakfast.

Nutrition: calories 519, fat 32.4, fiber 11, carbs 43.3, protein 19.1

Garbanzo Bean Salad

Preparation time: 10 minutes
Cooking time: 0 minutes
Servings: 4
Ingredients:

- 1 and ½ cups cucumber, cubed
- 15 ounces canned garbanzo beans, drained and rinsed
- 3 ounces black olives, pitted and sliced
- 1 tomato, chopped
- ¼ cup red onion, chopped
- 5 cups salad greens
- A pinch of salt and black pepper
- ½ cup feta cheese, crumbled
- 3 tablespoons olive oil
- 1 tablespoon lemon juice
- ¼ cup parsley, chopped

Directions:

1.   In a salad bowl, combine the garbanzo beans with the cucumber, tomato and the rest of the ingredients except the cheese and toss.

2.   Divide the mix into small bowls, sprinkle the cheese on top and serve for breakfast.

Nutrition: calories 268, fat 16, fiber 7, carbs 24, protein 9

Corn and Shrimp Salad

Preparation time: 10 minutes
Cooking time: 10 minutes
Servings: 4
Ingredients:

- 4 ears of sweet corn, husked
- 1 avocado, peeled, pitted and chopped
- ½ cup basil, chopped
- A pinch of salt and black pepper
- 1 pound shrimp, peeled and deveined
- 1 and ½ cups cherry tomatoes, halved
- ¼ cup olive oil

Directions:

1.   Put the corn in a pot, add water to cover, bring to a boil over medium heat, cook for 6 minutes, drain, cool down, cut corn from the cob and put it in a bowl.

2.   Thread the shrimp onto skewers and brush with some of the oil.

3.   Place the skewers on the preheated grill, cook over medium heat for 2 minutes on each side, remove from skewers and add over the corn.

4.   Add the rest of the ingredients to the bowl, toss, divide between plates and serve for breakfast.

Nutrition: calories 371, fat 22, fiber 5, carbs 25, protein 23

Tomato and Lentils Salad

Preparation time: 10 minutes
Cooking time: 35 minutes
Servings: 4
Ingredients:

- 2 yellow onions, chopped
- 4 garlic cloves, minced
- 2 cups brown lentils
- 1 tablespoon olive oil
- A pinch of salt and black pepper
- ½ teaspoon sweet paprika
- ½ teaspoon ginger, grated
- 3 cups water
- ¼ cup lemon juice
- ¾ cup Greek yogurt
- 3 tablespoons tomato paste

Directions:

1.   Heat up a pot with the oil over medium-high heat, add the onions and sauté for 2 minutes.

2.   Add the garlic and the lentils, stir and cook for 1 minute more.

3.   Add the water, bring to a simmer and cook covered for 30 minutes.

4.   Add the lemon juice and the remaining ingredients except the yogurt. toss, divide the mix into bowls, top with the yogurt and serve.

Nutrition: calories 294, fat 3, fiber 8, carbs 49, protein 21

Couscous and Chickpeas Bowls

Preparation time: 10 minutes
Cooking time: 6 minutes
Servings: 4
Ingredients:

- ¾ cup whole wheat couscous
- 1 yellow onion, chopped
- 1 tablespoon olive oil
- 1 cup water
- 2 garlic cloves, minced
- 15 ounces canned chickpeas, drained and rinsed
- A pinch of salt and black pepper
- 15 ounces canned tomatoes, chopped
- 14 ounces canned artichokes, drained and chopped
- ½ cup Greek olives, pitted and chopped
- ½ teaspoon oregano, dried
- 1 tablespoon lemon juice

Directions:
1. Put the water in a pot, bring to a boil over medium heat, add the couscous, stir, take off the heat, cover the pan, leave aside for 10 minutes and fluff with a fork.
2. Heat up a pan with the oil over medium-high heat, add the onion and sauté for 2 minutes.
3. Add the rest of the ingredients, toss and cook for 4 minutes more.
4. Add the couscous, toss, divide into bowls and serve for breakfast.

Nutrition: calories 340, fat 10, fiber 9, carbs 51, protein 11

Zucchini and Quinoa Pan

Preparation time: 10 minutes
Cooking time: 20 minutes
Servings: 4
Ingredients:
- 1 tablespoon olive oil
- 2 garlic cloves, minced
- 1 cup quinoa
- 1 zucchini, roughly cubed
- 2 tablespoons basil, chopped
- ¼ cup green olives, pitted and chopped
- 1 tomato, cubed
- ½ cup feta cheese, crumbled
- 2 cups water
- 1 cup canned garbanzo beans, drained and rinsed
- A pinch of salt and black pepper

Directions:
1. Heat up a pan with the oil over medium-high heat, add the garlic and quinoa and brown for 3 minutes.
2. Add the water, zucchinis, salt and pepper, toss, bring to a simmer and cook for 15 minutes.
3. Add the rest of the ingredients, toss, divide everything between plates and serve for breakfast.

Nutrition: calories 310, fat 11, fiber 6, carbs 42, protein 11

Orzo and Veggie Bowls

Preparation time: 10 minutes
Cooking time: 0 minutes
Servings: 4

Ingredients:
- 2 and ½ cups whole-wheat orzo, cooked
- 14 ounces canned cannellini beans, drained and rinsed
- 1 yellow bell pepper, cubed
- 1 green bell pepper, cubed
- A pinch of salt and black pepper
- 3 tomatoes, cubed
- 1 red onion, chopped
- 1 cup mint, chopped
- 2 cups feta cheese, crumbled
- 2 tablespoons olive oil
- ¼ cup lemon juice
- 1 tablespoon lemon zest, grated
- 1 cucumber, cubed
- 1 and ¼ cup kalamata olives, pitted and sliced
- 3 garlic cloves, minced

Directions:
1. In a salad bowl, combine the orzo with the beans, bell peppers and the rest of the ingredients, toss, divide the mix between plates and serve for breakfast.

Nutrition: calories 411, fat 17, fiber 13, carbs 51, protein 14

Lemon Peas Quinoa Mix

Preparation time: 10 minutes
Cooking time: 20 minutes
Servings: 4
Ingredients:
- 1 and ½ cups quinoa, rinsed
- 1 pound asparagus, steamed and chopped
- 3 cups water
- 2 tablespoons parsley, chopped
- 2 tablespoons lemon juice
- 1 teaspoon lemon zest, grated
- ½ pound sugar snap peas, steamed
- ½ pound green beans, trimmed and halved
- A pinch of salt and black pepper
- 3 tablespoons pumpkin seeds
- 1 cup cherry tomatoes, halved
- 2 tablespoons olive oil

Directions:
1. Put the water in a pot, bring to a boil over medium heat, add the quinoa, stir and simmer for 20 minutes.
2. Stir the quinoa, add the parsley, lemon juice and the rest of the ingredients, toss, divide between plates and serve for breakfast.

Nutrition: calories 417, fat 15, fiber 9, carbs 58, protein 16

Brown Rice Salad

Preparation time: 10 minutes
Cooking time: 0 minutes
Servings: 4
Ingredients:
- 9 ounces brown rice, cooked
- 7 cups baby arugula

- 15 ounces canned garbanzo beans, drained and rinsed
- 4 ounces feta cheese, crumbled
- ¾ cup basil, chopped
- A pinch of salt and black pepper
- 2 tablespoons lemon juice
- ¼ teaspoon lemon zest, grated
- ¼ cup olive oil

Directions:
1. In a salad bowl, combine the brown rice with the arugula, the beans and the rest of the ingredients, toss and serve cold for breakfast.
Nutrition: calories 473, fat 22, fiber 7, carbs 53, protein 13

Walnuts Yogurt Mix
Preparation time: 10 minutes
Cooking time: 0 minutes
Servings: 6
Ingredients:
- 2 and ½ cups Greek yogurt
- 1 and ½ cups walnuts, chopped
- 1 teaspoon vanilla extract
- ¾ cup honey
- 2 teaspoons cinnamon powder

Directions:
1. In a bowl, combine the yogurt with the walnuts and the rest of the ingredients, toss, divide into smaller bowls and keep in the fridge for 10 minutes before serving for breakfast.
Nutrition: calories 388, fat 24.6, fiber 2.9, carbs 39.1, protein 10.2

Tahini Pine Nuts Toast
Preparation time: 5 minutes
Cooking time: 0 minutes
Servings: 2
Ingredients:
- 2 whole wheat bread slices, toasted
- 1 teaspoon water
- 1 tablespoon tahini paste
- 2 teaspoons feta cheese, crumbled
- Juice of ½ lemon
- 2 teaspoons pine nuts
- A pinch of black pepper

Directions:
1. In a bowl, mix the tahini with the water and the lemon juice, whisk really well and spread over the toasted bread slices.
2. Top each serving with the remaining ingredients and serve for breakfast.
Nutrition: calories 142, fat 7.6, fiber 2.7, carbs 13.7, protein 5.8

Cheesy Olives Bread
Preparation time: 1 hour and 40 minutes
Cooking time: 30 minutes
Servings: 10
Ingredients:
- 4 cups whole-wheat flour

- 3 tablespoons oregano, chopped
- 2 teaspoons dry yeast
- ¼ cup olive oil
- 1 and ½ cups black olives, pitted and sliced
- 1 cup water
- ½ cup feta cheese, crumbled

Directions:
1. In a bowl, mix the flour with the water, the yeast and the oil, stir and knead your dough very well.
2. Put the dough in a bowl, cover with plastic wrap and keep in a warm place for 1 hour.
3. Divide the dough into 2 bowls and stretch each ball really well.
4. Add the rest of the ingredients on each ball and tuck them inside well kneading the dough again.
5. Flatten the balls a bit and leave them aside for 40 minutes more.
6. Transfer the balls to a baking sheet lined with parchment paper, make a small slit in each and bake at 425 degrees F for 30 minutes.
7. Serve the bread as a Mediterranean breakfast.
Nutrition: calories 251, fat 7.3, fiber 2.1, carbs 39.7, protein 6.7

Sweet Potato Tart
Preparation time: 10 minutes
Cooking time: 1 hour and 10 minutes
Servings: 8
Ingredients:
- 2 pounds sweet potatoes, peeled and cubed
- ¼ cup olive oil+ a drizzle
- 7 ounces feta cheese, crumbled
- 1 yellow onion, chopped
- 2 eggs, whisked
- ¼ cup almond milk
- 1 tablespoon herbs de Provence
- A pinch of salt and black pepper
- 6 phyllo sheets
- 1 tablespoon parmesan, grated

Directions:
1. In a bowl, combine the potatoes with half of the oil, salt and pepper, toss, spread on a baking sheet lined with parchment paper and roast at 400 degrees F for 25 minutes.
2. Meanwhile, heat up a pan with half of the remaining oil over medium heat, add the onion and sauté for 5 minutes.
3. In a bowl, combine the eggs with the milk, feta, herbs, salt, pepper, the onion, sweet potatoes and the rest of the oil and toss.
4. Arrange the phyllo sheets in a tart pan and brush them with a drizzle of oil.
5. Add the sweet potato mix and spread it well into the pan.
6. Sprinkle the parmesan on top and bake covered with tin foil at 350 degrees F for 20 minutes.
7. Remove the tin foil, bake the tart for 20 minutes more, cool it down, slice and serve for breakfast.
Nutrition: calories 476, fat 16.8, fiber 10.2, carbs 68.8, protein 13.9

Stuffed Pita Breads

Preparation time: 5 minutes
Cooking time: 15 minutes
Servings: 4
Ingredients:
- 1 and ½ tablespoons olive oil
- 1 tomato, cubed
- 1 garlic clove, minced
- 1 red onion, chopped
- ¼ cup parsley, chopped
- 15 ounces canned fava beans, drained and rinsed
- ¼ cup lemon juice
- Salt and black pepper to the taste
- 4 whole wheat pita bread pockets

Directions:
1. Heat up a pan with the oil over medium heat, add the onion, stir and sauté for 5 minutes.
2. Add the rest of the ingredients, stir and cook for 10 minutes more
3. Stuff the pita pockets with this mix and serve for breakfast.

Nutrition: calories 382, fat 1.8, fiber 27.6, carbs 66, protein 28.5

Blueberries Quinoa

Preparation time: 5 minutes
Cooking time: 0 minutes
Servings: 4
Ingredients:
- 2 cups almond milk
- 2 cups quinoa, already cooked
- ½ teaspoon cinnamon powder
- 1 tablespoon honey
- 1 cup blueberries
- ¼ cup walnuts, chopped

Directions:
1. In a bowl, mix the quinoa with the milk and the rest of the ingredients, toss, divide into smaller bowls and serve for breakfast.

Nutrition: calories 284, fat 14.3, fiber 3.2, carbs 15.4, protein 4.4

Endives, Fennel and Orange Salad

Preparation time: 5 minutes
Cooking time: 0 minutes
Servings: 4
Ingredients:
- 1 tablespoon balsamic vinegar
- 2 garlic cloves, minced
- 1 teaspoon Dijon mustard
- 2 tablespoons olive oil
- 1 tablespoon lemon juice
- Sea salt and black pepper to the taste
- ½ cup black olives, pitted and chopped
- 1 tablespoon parsley, chopped
- 7 cups baby spinach
- 2 endives, shredded
- 3 medium navel oranges, peeled and cut into segments

- 2 bulbs fennel, shredded

Directions:
1. In a salad bowl, combine the spinach with the endives, oranges, fennel and the rest of the ingredients, toss and serve for breakfast.

Nutrition: calories 97, fat 9.1, fiber 1.8, carbs 3.7, protein 1.9

Raspberries and Yogurt Smoothie

Preparation time: 5 minutes
Cooking time: 0 minutes
Servings: 2
Ingredients:
- 2 cups raspberries
- ½ cup Greek yogurt
- ½ cup almond milk
- ½ teaspoon vanilla extract

Directions:
1. In your blender, combine the raspberries with the milk, vanilla and the yogurt, pulse well, divide into 2 glasses and serve for breakfast.

Nutrition: calories 245, fat 9.5, fiber 2.3, carbs 5.6, protein 1.6

Farro Salad

Preparation time: 5 minutes
Cooking time: 4 minutes
Servings: 2
Ingredients:
- 1 tablespoon olive oil
- A pinch of salt and black pepper
- 1 bunch baby spinach, chopped
- 1 avocado, pitted, peeled and chopped
- 1 garlic clove, minced
- 2 cups farro, already cooked
- ½ cup cherry tomatoes, cubed

Directions:
1. Heat up a pan with the oil over medium heat, add the spinach, and the rest of the ingredients, toss, cook for 4 minutes, divide into bowls and serve.

Nutrition: calories 157, fat 13.7, fiber 5.5, carbs 8.6, protein 3.6

Cranberry and Dates Squares

Preparation time: 30 minutes
Cooking time: 0 minutes
Servings: 10
Ingredients:
- 12 dates, pitted and chopped
- 1 teaspoon vanilla extract
- ¼ cup honey
- ½ cup rolled oats
- ¾ cup cranberries, dried
- ¼ cup almond avocado oil, melted
- 1 cup walnuts, roasted and chopped
- ¼ cup pumpkin seeds

Directions:
1. In a bowl, mix the dates with the vanilla, honey and the rest of the ingredients, stir well and press

everything on a baking sheet lined with parchment paper.
2. Keep in the freezer for 30 minutes, cut into 10 squares and serve for breakfast.
Nutrition: calories 263, fat 13.4, fiber 4.7, carbs 14.3, protein 3.5

Cheesy Eggs Ramekins

Preparation time: 10 minutes
Cooking time: 10 minutes
Servings: 2
Ingredients:
- 1 tablespoon chives, chopped
- 1 tablespoon dill, chopped
- A pinch of salt and black pepper
- 2 tablespoons cheddar cheese, grated
- 1 tomato, chopped
- 2 eggs, whisked
- Cooking spray

Directions:
1. In a bowl, mix the eggs with the tomato and the rest of the ingredients except the cooking spray and whisk well.
2. Grease 2 ramekins with the cooking spray, divide the mix into each ramekin, bake at 400 degrees F for 10 minutes and serve.
Nutrition: calories 104, fat 7.1, fiber 0.6, carbs 2.6, protein 7.9

Potato and Pancetta Bowls

Preparation time: 10 minutes
Cooking time: 1 hour and 5 minutes
Servings: 4
Ingredients:
- 1 pound sweet potatoes, peeled and cut into small wedges
- 1 red onion, chopped
- 3 ounces pancetta, chopped
- 2 garlic cloves, minced
- 2 tablespoons olive oil
- 2 eggs, whisked
- 2 ounces goat cheese, crumbled
- 1 tablespoon parsley, chopped
- A pinch of salt and black pepper

Directions:
1. Put potatoes in a pot, add water to cover, add salt and pepper, bring to a boil over medium heat, simmer for 15 minutes, drain and put them in a bowl.
2. Heat up a pan with half of the oil over medium heat, add the onion, the potatoes, the eggs and the rest of the ingredients, toss and cook for 15 minutes.
3. Divide between plates and serve for breakfast.
Nutrition: calories

Cottage Cheese and Berries Omelet

Preparation time: 5 minutes
Cooking time: 4 minutes
Servings: 1
Ingredients:
- 1 egg, whisked

- ½ teaspoon olive oil
- 1 teaspoon cinnamon powder
- 1 tablespoon almond milk
- 3 ounces cottage cheese
- 4 ounces blueberries

Directions:
1. In a bowl, mix the egg with the rest of the ingredients except the oil and toss.
2. Heat up a pan with the oil over medium heat, add the eggs mix, spread, cook for 2 minutes on each side, transfer to a plate and serve.
Nutrition: calories

Salmon Frittata

Preparation time: 5 minutes
Cooking time: 27 minutes
Servings: 4
Ingredients:
- 1 pound gold potatoes, roughly cubed
- 1 tablespoon olive oil
- Cooking spray
- 2 salmon fillets, skinless and boneless
- 8 eggs, whisked
- 1 teaspoon mint, chopped
- A pinch of salt and black pepper

Directions:
1. Put the potatoes in a pot, add water to cover, bring to a boil over medium heat, cook for 12 minutes, drain and transfer to a bowl.
2. Arrange the salmon on a baking sheet lined with parchment paper, grease with cooking spray, broil over medium-high heat for 5 minutes on each side, cool down, flake and put in a separate bowl.
3. Heat up a pan with the oil over medium heat, add the potatoes, salmon, and the rest of the ingredients except the eggs and toss.
4. Add the eggs on top, put the lid on and cook over medium heat for 10 minutes.
5. Divide the salmon between plates and serve.
Nutrition: calories

Coriander Mushroom Salad

Preparation time: 5 minutes
Cooking time: 7 minutes
Servings: 6
Ingredients:
- ½ pounds white mushrooms, sliced
- 1 tablespoon olive oil
- 3 garlic cloves, minced
- Salt and black pepper to the taste
- 1 tomato, diced
- 1 avocado, peeled, pitted and cubed
- 3 tablespoons lime juice
- ½ cup chicken stock
- 2 tablespoons coriander, chopped

Directions:
1. Heat up a pan with the oil over medium heat, add the mushrooms and sauté them for 4 minutes.

2. Add the rest of the ingredients, toss, cook for 3-4 minutes more, divide into bowls and serve for breakfast.
Nutrition: calories

Cinnamon Apple and Lentils Porridge

Preparation time: 5 minutes
Cooking time: 10 minutes
Servings: 4
Ingredients:
- ½ cup walnuts, chopped
- 2 green apples, cored, peeled and cubed
- 3 tablespoons maple syrup
- 3 cups almond milk
- ½ cup red lentils
- ½ teaspoon cinnamon powder
- ½ cup cranberries, dried
- 1 teaspoon vanilla extract

Directions:
1. Put the milk in a pot, heat it up over medium heat, add the walnuts, apples, maple syrup and the rest of the ingredients, toss, simmer for 10 minutes, divide into bowls and serve.
Nutrition: calories 150, fat 2, fiber 1, carbs 3, protein 5

Lentils and Cheddar Frittata

Preparation time: 10 minutes
Cooking time: 15 minutes
Servings: 4
Ingredients:
- 1 red onion, chopped
- 2 tablespoons olive oil
- 1 cup sweet potatoes, boiled and chopped
- ¾ cup ham, chopped
- 4 eggs, whisked
- ¾ cup lentils, cooked
- 2 tablespoons Greek yogurt
- Salt and black pepper to the taste
- ½ cup cherry tomatoes, halved
- ¾ cup cheddar cheese, grated

Directions:
1. Heat up a pan with the oil over medium heat, add the onion, stir and sauté for 2 minutes.
2. Add the rest of the ingredients except the eggs and the cheese, toss and cook for 3 minutes more.
3. Add the eggs, sprinkle the cheese on top, cover the pan and cook for 10 minutes more.
4. Slice the frittata, divide between plates and serve.
Nutrition: calories 274, fat 17.3, fiber 3.5, carbs 8.9, protein 11.4

Seeds and Lentils Oats

Preparation time: 10 minutes
Cooking time: 50 minutes
Servings: 4
Ingredients:
- ½ cup red lentils

- ¼ cup pumpkin seeds, toasted
- 2 teaspoons olive oil
- ¼ cup rolled oats
- ¼ cup coconut flesh, shredded
- 1 tablespoon honey
- 1 tablespoon orange zest, grated
- 1 cup Greek yogurt
- 1 cup blackberries

Directions:
1. Spread the lentils on a baking sheet lined with parchment paper, introduce in the oven and roast at 370 degrees F for 30 minutes.
2. Add the rest of the ingredients except the yogurt and the berries, toss and bake at 370 degrees F for 20 minutes more.
3. Transfer this to a bowl, add the rest of the ingredients, toss, divide into smaller bowls and serve for breakfast.
Nutrition: calories 204, fat 7.1, fiber 10.4, carbs 27.6, protein 9.5

Tuna and Cheese Bake

Preparation time: 5 minutes
Cooking time: 15 minutes
Servings: 4
Ingredients:
- 10 ounces canned tuna, drained and flaked
- 4 eggs, whisked
- ½ cup feta cheese, shredded
- 1 tablespoon chives, chopped
- 1 tablespoon parsley, chopped
- Salt and black pepper to the taste
- 3 teaspoons olive oil

Directions:
1. Grease a baking dish with the oil, add the tuna and the rest of the ingredients except the cheese, toss and bake at 370 degrees F for 15 minutes.
2. Sprinkle the cheese on top, leave the mix aside for 5 minutes, slice and serve for breakfast.
Nutrition: calories 283, fat 14.2, fiber 5.6, carbs 12.1, protein 6.4

Tuna Sandwich

Preparation time: 5 minutes
Cooking time: 0 minutes
Servings: 2
Ingredients:
- 6 ounces canned tuna, drained and flaked
- 1 avocado, peeled, pitted and mashed
- 4 whole wheat bread slices
- A pinch of salt and black pepper
- 1 cup baby spinach
- 1 tablespoon feta cheese, crumbled

Directions:
1. In a bowl, mix the tuna with the cheese, salt and pepper and stir well.
2. Spread the mashed avocado on the bread slices, divide the tuna mix on 2 of them, divide the spinach as well, top with the other 2 slices and serve for breakfast.

Nutrition: calories 283, fat 11.2, fiber 3.4, carbs 9.8, protein 4.5

Yogurt Figs Mix

Preparation time: 5 minutes
Cooking time: 5 minutes
Servings: 4
Ingredients:
- 8 ounces figs, chopped
- 2 cups Greek yogurt
- 1 tablespoon honey
- 1 teaspoon cinnamon powder
- 1 tablespoon almonds, chopped
- 1 tablespoon walnuts, chopped
- ¼ cup pistachios, chopped

Directions:
1. Heat up a pan over medium heat, add the figs and the rest of the ingredients except the yogurt, stir and cook for 5 minutes.
2. Divide the yogurt into bowls, divide the figs mix on top, toss gently and serve.
Nutrition: calories 198, fat 4.2, fiber 6.3, carbs 42.1, protein 3.4

Mango and Spinach Bowls

Preparation time: 5 minutes
Cooking time: 0 minutes
Servings: 4

Ingredients:
- 1 cup baby arugula
- 1 cup baby spinach, chopped
- 1 mango, peeled and cubed
- 1 cup strawberries, halved
- 1 tablespoon hemp seeds
- 1 cucumber, sliced
- 1 tablespoon lime juice
- 1 tablespoon tahini paste
- 1 tablespoon water

Directions:
1. In a salad bowl, mix the arugula with the rest of the ingredients except the tahini and the water and toss.
2. In a small bowl, combine the tahini with the water, whisk well, add to the salad, toss, divide into small bowls and serve for breakfast.
Nutrition: calories 211, fat 4.5, fiber 6.5, carbs 10.2, protein 3.5

Oregano Quinoa and Spinach Muffins

Preparation time: 10 minutes
Cooking time: 35 minutes
Servings: 6
Ingredients:
- 1 cup quinoa
- 2 cups water
- 1 cup spinach, torn
- 2 spring onions, chopped
- 2 eggs, whisked
- ¼ cup parmesan cheese, grated

- ½ teaspoon garlic powder
- Sea salt and black pepper to the taste
- 2 teaspoons oregano, dried
- Cooking spray

Directions:
1. Put the water in a pan, heat up over medium heat, add the quinoa, bring to a simmer, cook for 10 minutes, take off the heat, fluff with a fork and transfer to a bowl.
2. Add the rest of the ingredients except the cooking spray and stir well.
3. Grease a muffin tin with the cooking spray, divide the quinoa and spinach mix, introduce in the oven at 350 degrees F and bake for 25 minutes.
4. Serve the muffins warm for breakfast.
Nutrition: calories 267, fat 11.2, fiber 2.3, carbs 8.5, protein 4.5

Apricots Couscous

Preparation time: 15 minutes
Cooking time: 4 minutes
Servings: 4
Ingredients:
- 3 cups almond milk
- 1 teaspoon cinnamon powder
- 1 cup apricots, chopped
- 1 cup couscous, uncooked
- 3 teaspoons honey
- 4 teaspoons avocado oil

Directions:
1. Heat up a pan with the milk over medium heat, add the cinnamon and the rest of the ingredients, toss, and simmer for 4 minutes.
2. Divide the mix into bowls, leave aside for 15 minutes and serve for breakfast,
Nutrition: calories 617, fat 44, fiber 7.1, carbs 52.3, protein 10.2

Tapioca Pudding

Preparation time: 30 minutes
Cooking time: 15 minutes
Servings: 3
Ingredients:
- ¼ cup pearl tapioca
- ¼ cup maple syrup
- 2 cups almond milk
- ½ cup coconut flesh, shredded
- 1 and ½ teaspoon lemon juice

Directions:
1. In a pan, combine the milk with the tapioca and the rest of the ingredients, bring to a simmer over medium heat, and cook for 15 minutes.
2. Divide the mix into bowls, cool it down and serve for breakfast.
Nutrition: calories 361, fat 28.5, fiber 2.7, carbs 28.3, protein 2.8

Greek Beans Tortillas

Preparation time: 5 minutes
Cooking time: 20 minutes
Servings: 4

Ingredients:
- 1 red onion, chopped
- 2 garlic cloves, minced
- 1 tablespoon olive oil
- 1 green bell pepper, sliced
- 3 cups canned pinto beans, drained and rinsed
- 2 red chili peppers, chopped
- 4 tablespoon parsley, chopped
- 1 teaspoon cumin, ground
- A pinch of salt and black pepper
- 4 whole wheat Greek tortillas
- 1 cup cheddar cheese, shredded

Directions:
1. Heat up a pan with the oil over medium heat, add the onion and sauté for 5 minutes.
2. Add the rest of the ingredients except the tortillas and the cheese, stir and cook for 15 minutes.
3. Divide this beans mix on each Greek tortilla, also divide the cheese, roll the tortillas and serve for breakfast.

Nutrition: calories 673, fat 14.9, fiber 23.7, carbs 75.4, protein 39

Baked Cauliflower Hash

Preparation time: 10 minutes
Cooking time: 25 minutes
Servings: 4
Ingredients:
- 4 cups cauliflower florets
- 1 tablespoon olive oil
- 2 cups white mushrooms, sliced
- 1 cup cherry tomatoes, halved
- 1 yellow onion, chopped
- 2 garlic cloves, minced
- ¼ teaspoon garlic powder
- 3 tablespoons basil, chopped
- 3 tablespoons mint, chopped
- 1 tablespoon dill, chopped

Directions:
1. Spread the cauliflower florets on a baking sheet lined with parchment paper, add the rest of the ingredients, introduce in the oven at 350 degrees F and bake for 25 minutes.
2. Divide the hash between plates and serve for breakfast.

Nutrition: calories 367, fat 14.3, fiber 3.5, carbs 16.8, protein 12.2

Eggs, Mint and Tomatoes

Preparation time: 10 minutes
Cooking time: 15 minutes
Servings: 2
Ingredients:
- 2 eggs, whisked
- 2 tomatoes, cubed
- 2 teaspoons olive oil
- 1 tablespoon mint, chopped
- 1 tablespoon chives, chopped
- Salt and black pepper to the taste

Directions:
1. Heat up a pan with the oil over medium heat, add the tomatoes and the rest of the ingredients except the eggs, stir and cook for 5 minutes.
2. Add the eggs, toss, cook for 10 minutes more, divide between plates and serve.

Nutrition: calories 300, fat 15.3, fiber 4.5, carbs 17.7, protein 11

Bacon, Spinach and Tomato Sandwich

Preparation time: 5 minutes
Cooking time: 0 minutes
Servings: 1
Ingredients:
- 2 whole-wheat bread slices, toasted
- 1 tablespoon Dijon mustard
- 3 bacon slices
- Salt and black pepper to the taste
- 2 tomato slices
- ¼ cup baby spinach

Directions:
1. Spread the mustard on each bread slice, divide the bacon and the rest of the ingredients on one slice, top with the other one, cut in half and serve for breakfast.

Nutrition: calories 246, fat 11.2, fiber 4.5, carbs 17.5, protein 8.3

Veggie Salad

Preparation time: 5 minutes
Cooking time: 0 minutes
Servings: 4
Ingredients:
- 2 tomatoes, cut into wedges
- 2 red bell peppers, chopped
- 1 cucumber, chopped
- 1 red onion, sliced
- ½ cup kalamata olives, pitted and sliced
- 2 ounces feta cheese, crumbled
- ¼ cup lime juice
- ½ cup olive oil
- 2 garlic cloves, minced
- 1 tablespoon oregano, chopped
- Salt and black pepper to the taste

Directions:
1. In a large salad bowl, combine the tomatoes with the peppers and the rest of the ingredients except the cheese and toss.
2. Divide the salad into smaller bowls, sprinkle the cheese on top and serve for breakfast.

Nutrition: calories 327, fat 11.2, fiber 4.4, carbs 16.7, protein 6.4

Salmon and Bulgur Salad

Preparation time: 25 minutes
Cooking time: 10 minutes
Servings: 4
Ingredients:
- 1 pound salmon fillet, skinless and boneless
- 1 tablespoon olive oil

- 1 cup bulgur
- 1 cup parsley, chopped
- ¼ cup mint, chopped
- 3 tablespoons lemon juice
- 1 red onion, sliced
- Salt and black pepper to the taste
- 2 cup hot water

Directions:
1. Heat up a pan with half of the oil over medium heat, add the salmon, some salt and pepper, cook for 5 minutes on each side, cool down, flake and put in a salad bowl.
2. In another bowl, mix the bulgur with hot water, cover, leave aside for 25 minutes, drain and transfer to the bowl with the salmon.
3. Add the rest of the ingredients, toss and serve for breakfast.

Nutrition: calories 321, fat 11.3, fiber 7.9, carbs 30.8, protein 27.6

Herbed Quinoa and Asparagus

Preparation time: 10 minutes
Cooking time: 0 minutes
Servings: 4
Ingredients:
- 3 cups asparagus, steamed and roughly chopped
- 1 tablespoon olive oil
- 3 tablespoons balsamic vinegar
- 1 and ¾ cups quinoa, cooked
- 2 teaspoons mustard
- Salt and black pepper to the taste
- 5 ounces baby spinach
- ½ cup parsley, chopped
- 1 tablespoon thyme, chopped
- 1 tablespoon tarragon, chopped

Directions:
1. In a salad bowl, combine the asparagus with the quinoa, spinach and the rest of the ingredients, toss and keep in the fridge for 10 minutes before serving for breakfast.

Nutrition: calories 323, fat 11.3, fiber 3.4, carbs 16.4, protein 10

Lettuce and Strawberry Salad

Preparation time: 5 minutes
Cooking time: 0 minutes
Servings: 6
Ingredients:
- 1 avocado, peeled, pitted and mashed
- 2 tablespoons almond milk
- 1 tablespoon poppy seeds
- 4 cups romaine lettuce leaves, torn
- 1 tablespoon balsamic vinegar
- 1 cup strawberries, sliced
- 2 tablespoons almonds, toasted and chopped

Directions:
1. In a bowl, mix the avocado with the lettuce and the rest of the ingredients, toss and serve for breakfast,

Nutrition: calories 145, fat 1.9, fiber 1.2, carbs 3.6, protein 2.3

Lunch Recipes

Tomato and Halloumi Platter

Preparation time: 5 minutes
Cooking time: 4 minutes
Servings: 4
Ingredients:
- 1 pound tomatoes, sliced
- ½ pound halloumi, cut into 4 slices
- 2 tablespoons parsley, chopped
- 1 tablespoon basil, chopped
- 2 tablespoons olive oil
- A pinch of salt and black pepper
- Juice of 1 lemon

Directions:
1. Brush the halloumi slices with half of the oil, put them on your preheated grill and cook over medium-high heat and cook for 2 minutes on each side.
2. Arrange the tomato slices on a platter, season with salt and pepper, drizzle the lemon juice and the rest of the oil all over, top with the halloumi slices, sprinkle the herbs on top and serve for lunch.

Nutrition: calories 181, fat 7.3, fiber 1.4, carbs 4.6, protein 1.1

Chickpeas and Millet Stew

Preparation time: 10 minutes
Cooking time: 1 hour and 5 minutes
Servings: 4
Ingredients:
- 1 cup millet
- 2 tablespoons olive oil
- A pinch of salt and black pepper
- 1 eggplant, cubed
- 1 yellow onion, chopped
- 14 ounces canned tomatoes, chopped
- 14 ounces canned chickpeas, drained and rinsed
- 3 garlic cloves, minced
- 2 tablespoons harissa paste
- 1 bunch cilantro, chopped
- 2 cups water

Directions:
1. Put the water in a pan, bring to a simmer over medium heat, add the millet, simmer for 25 minutes, take off the heat, fluff with a fork and leave aside for now.
2. Heat up a pan with half of the oil over medium heat, add the eggplant, salt and pepper, stir, cook for 10 minutes and transfer to a bowl.
3. Add the rest of the oil to the pan, heat up over medium heat again, add the onion and sauté for 10 minutes.
4. Add the garlic, more salt and pepper, the harrisa, chickpeas, tomatoes and return the eggplant, stir and cook over low heat for 15 minutes more.
5. Add the millet, toss, divide the mix into bowls, sprinkle the cilantro on top and serve.

Nutrition: calories 671, fat 15.6, fiber 27.5, carbs 87.5, protein 27.1

Chicken Salad

Preparation time: 30 minutes
Cooking time: 45 minutes
Servings: 4
Ingredients:
- 1 and ½ pounds chicken breast, skinless, boneless
- 1 tablespoon dill, chopped
- Zest of 2 lemons, grated
- Juice of 2 lemons
- 3 tablespoons olive oil
- 1 tablespoon oregano, chopped
- 3 tablespoons parsley, chopped
- A pinch of salt and black pepper

For the barley:
- 2 and ½ cups chicken stock
- 1 cup barley
- 1 teaspoon oregano, dried
- Zest of 1 lemon, grated
- Juice of 1 lemon
- ¼ cup olive oil
- 2 red leaf lettuce heads, chopped
- 1 red onion, sliced
- 1 pint cherry tomatoes, sliced
- 2 avocados, peeled, pitted and sliced

Directions:
1. Put the chicken breasts in a bowl, add the dill, zest of 2 lemons, juice of 2 lemons, 3 tablespoons oil, 1 tablespoon oregano, parsley, salt and pepper, toss, cover the bowl and leave aside for 30 minutes.
2. Heat up your grill over medium-high heat, add the chicken, cook for 6 minutes on each side, cool down, slice and put in a bowl.
3. Put the stock in a pot, add the barley, salt and pepper, bring to a simmer over medium heat, cook for 45 minutes, drain and put in the same bowl with the chicken.
4. Add the dried oregano, zest of 1 lemon, juice of 1 lemon, ¼ cup oil, the lettuce, onion, tomatoes and the avocados, toss and serve.

Nutrition: calories 342, fat 17.4, fiber 16.5, carbs 27.7, protein 26.9

Chicken Skillet

Preparation time: 10 minutes
Cooking time: 35 minutes
Servings: 6
Ingredients:
- 6 chicken thighs, bone-in and skin-on
- Juice of 2 lemons
- 1 teaspoon oregano, dried
- 1 red onion, chopped
- Salt and black pepper to the taste
- 1 teaspoon garlic powder
- 2 garlic cloves, minced
- 2 tablespoons olive oil
- 2 and ½ cups chicken stock

- 1 cup white rice
- 1 tablespoon oregano, chopped
- 1 cup green olives, pitted and sliced
- 1/3 cup parsley, chopped
- ½ cup feta cheese, crumbled

Directions:
1. Heat up a pan with the oil over medium heat, add the chicken thighs skin side down, cook for 4 minutes on each side and transfer to a plate.
2. Add the garlic and the onion to the pan, stir and sauté for 5 minutes.
3. Add the rice, salt, pepper, the stock, oregano, and lemon juice, stir, cook for 1-2 minutes more and take off the heat.
4. Add the chicken to the pan, introduce the pan in the oven and bake at 375 degrees F for 25 minutes.
5. Add the cheese, olives and the parsley, divide the whole mix between plates and serve for lunch.

Nutrition: calories 435, fat 18.5, fiber 13.6, carbs 27.8, protein 25.6

Tuna and Couscous

Preparation time: 10 minutes
Cooking time: 0 minutes
Servings: 4
Ingredients:
- 1 cup chicken stock
- 1 and ¼ cups couscous
- A pinch of salt and black pepper
- 10 ounces canned tuna, drained and flaked
- 1 pint cherry tomatoes, halved
- ½ cup pepperoncini, sliced
- 1/3 cup parsley, chopped
- 1 tablespoon olive oil
- ¼ cup capers, drained
- Juice of ½ lemon

Directions:
1. Put the stock in a pan, bring to a boil over medium-high heat, add the couscous, stir, take off the heat, cover, leave aside for 10 minutes, fluff with a fork and transfer to a bowl.
2. Add the tuna and the rest of the ingredients, toss and serve for lunch right away.

Nutrition: calories 253, fat 11.5, fiber 3.4, carbs 16.5, protein 23.2

Chicken Stuffed Peppers

Preparation time: 10 minutes
Cooking time: 0 minutes
Servings: 6
Ingredients:
- 1 cup Greek yogurt
- 2 tablespoons mustard
- Salt and black pepper to the taste
- 1 pound rotisserie chicken meat, cubed
- 4 celery stalks, chopped
- 2 tablespoons balsamic vinegar
- 1 bunch scallions, sliced
- ¼ cup parsley, chopped
- 1 cucumber, sliced

- 3 red bell peppers, halved and deseeded
- 1 pint cherry tomatoes, quartered

Directions:
1. In a bowl, mix the chicken with the celery and the rest of the ingredients except the bell peppers and toss well.
2. Stuff the peppers halves with the chicken mix and serve for lunch.

Nutrition: calories 266, fat 12.2, fiber 4.5, carbs 15.7, protein 3.7

Turkey Fritters and Sauce

Preparation time: 10 minutes
Cooking time: 30 minutes
Servings: 4
Ingredients:
- 2 garlic cloves, minced
- 1 egg
- 1 red onion, chopped
- 1 tablespoon olive oil
- ¼ teaspoon red pepper flakes
- 1 pound turkey meat, ground
- ½ teaspoon oregano, dried
- Cooking spray

For the sauce:
- 1 cup Greek yogurt
- 1 cucumber, chopped
- 1 tablespoon olive oil
- ¼ teaspoon garlic powder
- 2 tablespoons lemon juice
- ¼ cup parsley, chopped

Directions:
1. Heat up a pan with 1 tablespoon oil over medium heat, add the onion and the garlic, sauté for 5 minutes, cool down and transfer to a bowl.
2. Add the meat, turkey, oregano and pepper flakes, stir and shape medium fritters out of this mix.
3. Heat up another pan greased with cooking spray over medium-high heat, add the turkey fritters and brown for 5 minutes on each side.
4. Introduce the pan in the oven and bake the fritters at 375 degrees F for 15 minutes more.
5. Meanwhile, in a bowl, mix the yogurt with the cucumber, oil, garlic powder, lemon juice and parsley and whisk really well.
6. Divide the fritters between plates, spread the sauce all over and serve for lunch.

Nutrition: calories 364, fat 16.8, fiber 5.5, carbs 26.8, protein 23.4

Stuffed Eggplants

Preparation time: 10 minutes
Cooking time: 35 minutes
Servings: 4
Ingredients:
- 2 eggplants, halved lengthwise and 2/3 of the flesh scooped out
- 3 tablespoons olive oil
- 1 red onion, chopped
- 2 garlic cloves, minced

- 1 pint white mushrooms, sliced
- 2 cups kale, torn
- 2 cups quinoa, cooked
- 1 tablespoon thyme, chopped
- Zest and juice of 1 lemon
- Salt and black pepper to the taste
- ½ cup Greek yogurt
- 3 tablespoons parsley, chopped

Directions:
1. Rub the inside of each eggplant half with half of the oil and arrange them on a baking sheet lined with parchment paper.
2. Heat up a pan with the rest of the oil over medium heat, add the onion and the garlic and sauté for 5 minutes.
3. Add the mushrooms and cook for 5 minutes more.
4. Add the kale, salt, pepper, thyme, lemon zest and juice, stir, cook for 5 minutes more and take off the heat.
5. Stuff the eggplant halves with the mushroom mix, introduce them in the oven and bake 400 degrees F for 20 minutes.
6. Divide the eggplants between plates, sprinkle the parsley and the yogurt on top and serve for lunch.

Nutrition: calories 512, fat 16.4, fiber 17.5, carbs 78, protein 17.2

Salmon Bowls

Preparation time: 10 minutes
Cooking time: 40 minutes
Servings: 4
Ingredients:
- 2 cups farro
- Juice of 2 lemons
- 1/3 cup olive oil+ 2 tablespoons
- Salt and black pepper
- 1 cucumber, chopped
- ¼ cup balsamic vinegar
- 1 garlic cloves, minced
- ¼ cup parsley, chopped
- ¼ cup mint, chopped
- 2 tablespoons mustard
- 4 salmon fillets, boneless

Directions:
1. Put water in a large pot, bring to a boil over medium-high heat, add salt and the farro, stir, simmer for 30 minutes, drain, transfer to a bowl, add the lemon juice, mustard, garlic, salt, pepper and 1/3 cup oil, toss and leave aside for now.
2. In another bowl, mash the cucumber with a fork, add the vinegar, salt, pepper, the parsley, dill and mint and whisk well.
3. Heat up a pan with the rest of the oil over medium heat, add the salmon fillets skin side down, cook for 5 minutes on each side, cool them down and break into pieces.
4. Add over the farro, add the cucumber dressing, toss and serve for lunch.

Nutrition: calories 281, fat 12.7, fiber 1.7, carbs 5.8, protein 36.5

Spicy Potato Salad

Preparation time: 10 minutes
Cooking time: 15 minutes
Servings: 4
Ingredients:
- 1 and ½ pounds baby potatoes, peeled and halved
- A pinch of salt and black pepper
- 2 tablespoons harissa paste
- 6 ounces Greek yogurt
- Juice of 1 lemon
- ¼ cup red onion, chopped
- ¼ cup parsley, chopped

Directions:
1. Put the potatoes in a pot, add water to cover, add salt, bring to a boil over medium-high heat, cook for 12 minutes, drain and transfer them to a bowl.
2. Add the harissa and the rest of the ingredients, toss and serve for lunch.

Nutrition: calories 354, fat 19.2, fiber 4.5, carbs 24.7, protein 11.2

Chicken and Rice Soup

Preparation time: 10 minutes
Cooking time: 35 minutes
Servings: 4
Ingredients:
- 6 cups chicken stock
- 1 and ½ cups chicken meat, cooked and shredded
- 1 bay leaf
- 1 yellow onion, chopped
- 2 tablespoons olive oil
- 1/3 cup white rice
- 1 egg, whisked
- Juice of ½ lemon
- 1 cup asparagus, trimmed and halved
- 1 cup carrots, chopped
- ½ cup dill, chopped
- Salt and black pepper to the taste

Directions:
1. Heat up a pot with the oil over medium heat, add the onions and sauté for 5 minutes.
2. Add the stock, dill, the rice and the bay leaf, stir, bring to a boil over medium heat and cook for 10 minutes.
3. Add the rest of the ingredients except the egg and the lemon juice, stir and cook for 15 minutes more.
4. Add the egg whisked with the lemon juice gradually, whisk the soup, cook for 2 minutes more, divide into bowls an serve.

Nutrition: calories 263, fat 18.5, fiber 4.5, carbs 19.8, protein 14.5

Chicken and Carrots Soup

Preparation time: 10 minutes

Cooking time: 1 hour and 20 minutes
Servings: 6
Ingredients:
- 1 whole chicken, cut into medium pieces
- 3 carrots, sliced
- 4 eggs, whisked
- Juice of 2 lemons
- ¼ cup dill, chopped
- Salt and black pepper to the taste
- 8 cups water

Directions:
1. Put the chicken pieces in a pot, add the water, bring to a boil over medium heat, cover the pot and simmer for 1 hour.
2. Transfer the chicken to a plate, cool it down, discard bones, return the meat to the pot and heat it up again over medium heat.
3. Add the rest of the ingredients except the eggs, stir and simmer the soup for 10 minutes more.
4. Add the eggs mixed with 2 cups of stock, stir the soup, cook for 2-3 minutes more, divide into bowls and serve.

Nutrition: calories 264, fat 17.5, fiber 4.8, carbs 28.7, protein 16.3

Roasted Peppers Soup

Preparation time: 10 minutes
Cooking time: 55 minutes
Servings: 4
Ingredients:
- 2 tomatoes, halved
- 3 red bell peppers, halved and deseeded
- 1 yellow onion, quartered
- 2 garlic cloves, peeled and halved
- 2 tablespoons olive oil
- 2 cups veggie stock
- A pinch of salt and black pepper
- 2 tablespoons tomato paste
- ¼ cup parsley, chopped
- ¼ teaspoon Italian seasoning
- ¼ teaspoon sweet paprika

Directions:
1. Spread the bell peppers, tomatoes, onion and garlic on a baking sheet lined with parchment paper, add oil, salt and pepper and bake at 375 degrees F for 45 minutes.
2. Heat up a pot with the stock over medium heat, add the roasted vegetables and the rest of the ingredients, stir, bring to a simmer and cook for 10 minutes.
3. Blend the mix using an immersion blender, divide the soup into bowls and serve.

Nutrition: calories 273, fat 11.2, fiber 3.4, carbs 15.7, protein 5.6

Lentils Soup

Preparation time: 10 minutes
Cooking time: 45 minutes
Servings: 6
Ingredients:

- 1 yellow onion, chopped
- 2 tablespoons olive oil
- 2 celery stalks, chopped
- 1 carrot, sliced
- 1/3 cup parsley, chopped
- ½ cup cilantro, chopped
- 2 and ½ tablespoons garlic, minced
- 2 tablespoons ginger, grated
- 1 teaspoon turmeric powder
- 2 teaspoons sweet paprika
- 1 teaspoon cinnamon powder
- 1 and ¼ cups red lentils
- 15 ounces canned chickpeas, drained and rinsed
- 28 ounces canned tomatoes and juice, crushed
- 8 cups chicken stock
- A pinch of salt and black pepper

Directions:
1. Heat up a pot with the oil over medium heat, add the onion, ginger, garlic, celery and carrots and sauté for 5 minutes.
2. Add the rest of the ingredients, stir, bring to a simmer over medium heat and cook for 35 minutes.
3. Ladle the soup into bowls and serve right away.

Nutrition: calories 238, fat 7.3, fiber 6.3, carbs 32, protein 14

White Bean Soup

Preparation time: 10 minutes
Cooking time: 8 hours
Servings: 6
Ingredients:
- 1 cup celery, chopped
- 1 cup carrots, chopped
- 1 yellow onion, chopped
- 6 cups veggie stock
- 4 garlic cloves, minced
- 2 cup navy beans, dried
- ½ teaspoon basil, dried
- ½ teaspoon sage, dried
- 1 teaspoon thyme, dried
- A pinch of salt and black pepper

Directions:
1. In your slow cooker, combine the beans with the stock and the rest of the ingredients, put the lid on and cook on Low for 8 hours.
2. Divide the soup into bowls and serve right away.

Nutrition: calories 264, fat 17.5, fiber 4.5, carbs 23.7, protein 11.5

Veggie Soup

Preparation time: 10 minutes
Cooking time: 45 minutes
Servings: 8
Ingredients:
- 1 yellow onion, chopped
- 4 garlic cloves, minced
- ½ cup carrots, chopped
- 1 zucchini, chopped

- 1 yellow squash, peeled and cubed
- 2 tablespoons parsley, chopped
- 3 tablespoons olive oil
- ¼ cup celery, chopped
- 30 ounces canned cannellini beans, drained and rinsed
- 30 ounces canned red kidney beans, drained and rinsed
- 4 cups veggie stock
- 2 cups water
- ¼ teaspoon thyme, dried
- ½ teaspoon basil, dried
- A pinch of salt and black pepper
- 4 cups baby spinach
- ¼ cup parmesan, grated

Directions:
1.   Heat up a pot with the oil over medium heat, add the onion, garlic, carrots, squash, zucchini, parsley and the celery, stir and sauté for 5 minutes.
2.   Add the rest of the ingredients except the spinach and the parmesan, stir, bring to a simmer over medium heat and cook for 30 minutes.
3.   Add the spinach, cook the soup for 10 minutes more, divide into bowls, sprinkle the cheese on top and serve.
Nutrition: calories 300, fat 11.3, fiber 3.4, carbs 17.5, protein 10

Seafood Gumbo

Preparation time: 10 minutes
Cooking time: 30 minutes
Servings: 4
Ingredients:
- ¼ cup tapioca flour
- ¼ cup olive oil
- 1 cup celery, chopped
- 1 white onion, chopped
- 1 red bell pepper, chopped
- 1 green bell pepper, chopped
- 1 red chili, chopped
- 2 cups okra, chopped
- 2 garlic cloves, minced
- 1 cup canned tomatoes, crushed
- 1 teaspoon thyme, dried
- 2 cups fish stock
- 1 bay leaf
- 16 ounces canned crab meat, drained
- 1 pound shrimp, peeled and deveined
- ¼ cup parsley, chopped
- Salt and black pepper to the taste

Directions:
1.   Heat up a pot with the oil over medium heat, add the flour, whisk to obtain a paste and cook for about 5 minutes.
2.   Add the bell peppers, the onions, celery and the okra and sauté for 5 minutes.
3.   Add the rest of the ingredients except the crab, shrimp, and parsley, stir, bring to a simmer and cook for 15 minutes.

4.   Add the remaining ingredients, simmer the soup for 10 minutes more, divide into bowls and serve.
Nutrition: calories 363, fat 2, fiber 5, carbs 18, protein 40

Chicken and Orzo Soup

Preparation time: 10 minutes
Cooking time: 11 minutes
Servings: 4
Ingredients:
- ½ cup carrot, chopped
- 1 yellow onion, chopped
- 12 cups chicken stock
- 2 cups kale, chopped
- 3 cups chicken meat, cooked and shredded
- 1 cup orzo
- ¼ cup lemon juice
- 1 tablespoon olive oil

Directions:
1.   Heat up a pot with the oil over medium heat, add the onion and sauté for 3 minutes.
2.   Add the carrots and the rest of the ingredients, stir, bring to a simmer and cook for 8 minutes more.
3.   Ladle into bowls and serve hot.
Nutrition: calories 300, fat 12.2, fiber 5.4, carbs 16.5, protein 12.2

Lentils Soup

Preparation time: 10 minutes
Cooking time: 8 hours
Servings: 6
Ingredients:
- 2 cups red lentils, dried
- 1 yellow onion, chopped
- 2 celery stalks, chopped
- 2 carrots, sliced
- 3 garlic cloves, minced
- 15 ounces canned tomatoes, chopped
- 2 chipotle chili peppers, chopped
- 7 cups veggie stock
- 1 and ½ teaspoons cumin, ground
- Salt and black pepper to the taste
- 2 teaspoons adobo sauce
- ¼ cup cilantro, chopped
- 2 tablespoons lime juice

Directions:
1.   In your slow cooker, combine the lentils with the tomatoes, chili peppers and the rest of the ingredients except the cilantro and the lime juice, put the lid on and cook on Low for 8 hours.
2.   Add the cilantro and the lime juice, stir, ladle the soup into bowls and serve.
Nutrition: calories 276, fat 1, fiber 21, carbs 48, protein 17

Zucchini Soup

Preparation time: 10 minutes
Cooking time: 20 minutes
Servings: 8

Ingredients:
- 2 and ½ pounds zucchinis, roughly chopped
- 2 tablespoons olive oil
- 1 yellow onion, chopped
- 4 garlic cloves, minced
- 4 cups chicken stock
- ½ cup basil, chopped
- Salt and black pepper to the taste

Directions:
1. Heat up a pot with the oil over medium heat, add the zucchinis and the onion and sauté for 5 minutes.
2. Add the garlic and the rest of the ingredients except the basil, stir, bring to a simmer and cook for 15 minutes over medium heat.
3. Add the basil, blend the soup using an immersion blender, ladle into bowls and serve.

Nutrition: calories 182, fat 7.6, fiber 1.5, carbs 12.6, protein 2.3

Tuscan Soup

Preparation time: 10 minutes
Cooking time: 15 minutes
Servings: 6
Ingredients:
- 1 yellow onion, chopped
- 4 garlic cloves, minced
- 2 tablespoons olive oil
- ½ cup celery, chopped
- ½ cup carrots, chopped
- 15 ounces canned tomatoes, chopped
- 1 zucchini, chopped
- 6 cups veggie stock
- 2 tablespoons tomato paste
- 15 ounces canned white beans, drained and rinsed
- 2 handfuls baby spinach
- 1 tablespoon basil, chopped
- Salt and black pepper to the taste

Directions:
1. Heat up a pot with the oil over medium heat, add the garlic and the onion and sauté for 5 minutes.
2. Add the rest of the ingredients, stir, bring the soup to a simmer and cook for 10 minutes.
3. Ladle the soup into bowls and serve right away.

Nutrition: calories 471, fat 8.2, fiber 19.4, carbs 76.5, protein 27.6

Cauliflower Cream

Preparation time: 10 minutes
Cooking time: 1 hour and 10 minutes
Servings: 8
Ingredients:
- 1 cauliflower head, florets separated
- 1 teaspoon garlic powder
- 2 tablespoons olive oil
- 1 yellow onion, chopped
- Salt and black pepper to the taste
- 5 cups chicken stock
- 2 tablespoons garlic, minced

- 2 and ½ cups cheddar cheese, shredded

Directions:
1. Spread the cauliflower on a baking sheet lined with parchment paper, add garlic powder, half of the oil, salt and pepper and roast at 425 degrees F for 30 minutes.
2. Heat up a pot with the rest of the oil over medium heat, add the onion and sauté for 5 minutes.
3. Add the roasted cauliflower and the rest of the ingredients except the cheddar, stir and simmer the soup for 30 minutes.
4. Blend the soup using an immersion blender, add the cheese, stir, divide the soup into bowls and serve.

Nutrition: calories 243, fat 17, fiber 2.3, carbs 41.1, protein 13.7

White Beans and Orange Soup

Preparation time: 10 minutes
Cooking time: 37 minutes
Servings: 4
Ingredients:
- 1 yellow onion, chopped
- 5 celery sticks, chopped
- 4 carrots, chopped
- 1 cup olive oil
- ½ teaspoon oregano, dried
- 1 bay leaf
- 3 orange slices, peeled
- 30 ounces canned white beans, drained
- 2 tablespoons tomato paste
- 2 cups water
- 6 cups chicken stock

Directions:
1. Heat up a pot with the oil over medium heat, add the onion, celery, carrots, the bay leaf and the oregano, stir and sauté for 5 minutes.
2. Add the orange slices and cook for 2 minutes more.
3. Add the rest of the ingredients, stir, bring a simmer and cook over medium heat for 30 minutes.
4. Ladle the soup into bowls and serve.

Nutrition: calories 273, fat 16.3, fiber 8.4, carbs 15.6, protein 7.4

Basil Zucchini Soup

Preparation time: 10 minutes
Cooking time: 20 minutes
Servings: 4
Ingredients:
- 2 tablespoons olive oil
- 3 garlic cloves, minced
- 1 yellow onion, chopped
- 4 zucchinis, cubed
- 4 cups chicken stock
- Zest of 1 lemon, grated
- ½ cup basil, chopped
- Salt and black pepper to the taste

Directions:

1. Heat up a pot with the oil over medium heat, add the onion and the garlic and sauté for 5 minutes.
2. Add the zucchinis and the rest of the ingredients except the basil, bring to a simmer and cook over medium heat for 15 minutes.
3. Add the basil, stir, divide the soup into bowls and serve.
Nutrition: calories 274, fat 11.1, fiber 4.5, carbs 16.5, protein 4.5

Chicken and Leeks Soup

Preparation time: 10 minutes
Cooking time: 50 minutes
Servings: 6
Ingredients:
- 2 pounds chicken breast, skinless, boneless and cubed
- ½ cup olive oil
- 2 leeks, sliced
- 4 spring onions, chopped
- 1 small green cabbage head, shredded
- 4 celery sticks, chopped
- 4 cups veggie stock
- ½ teaspoon sweet paprika
- A pinch of nutmeg, ground
- Salt and black pepper to the taste

Directions:
1. Heat up a pot with the oil over medium-high heat, add the chicken and brown for 2 minutes on each side.
2. Add the leeks, onions and celery and sauté for 1 minute more.
3. Add the rest of the ingredients, bring to a simmer and cook over medium heat for 45 minutes.
4. Ladle the soup into bowls and serve.
Nutrition: calories 310, fat 15.3, fiber 8.7, carbs 24.6, protein 18.4

Lemony Lamb Soup

Preparation time: 10 minutes
Cooking time: 1 hour and 5 minutes
Servings: 4
Ingredients:
- ½ cup olive oil
- 2 pounds lamb meat, cubed
- 5 cups water
- 5 spring onions, chopped
- 2 tablespoons dill, chopped
- Juice of 2 lemons
- Salt and black pepper to the taste
- 3 eggs, whisked
- 1 cup baby spinach

Directions:
1. Heat up a pot with the oil over medium heat, add the lamb and brown for 10 minutes stirring from time to time.
2. Add the onions and sauté for 3 minutes more.
3. Add the water, salt and pepper, stir and simmer over medium heat for 30 minutes.

4. Add the spinach, eggs whisked with the lemon juice and some of the soup, whisk the soup well and cook for 20 minutes more.
5. Add the dill, stir, ladle the soup into bowls and serve.
Nutrition: calories 275, fat 28.5, fiber 1, carbs 2.8, protein 5

Sausage and Beans Soup

Preparation time: 10 minutes
Cooking time: 20 minutes
Servings: 4
Ingredients:
- 1 pound Italian pork sausage, sliced
- ¼ cup olive oil
- 1 carrot, chopped
- 1 yellow onion, chopped
- 1 celery stalk, chopped
- 2 garlic cloves, minced
- ½ pound kale, chopped
- 4 cups chicken stock
- 28 ounces canned cannellini beans, drained and rinsed
- 1 bay leaf
- 1 teaspoon rosemary, dried
- Salt and black pepper to the taste
- ½ cup parmesan, grated

Directions:
1. Heat up a pot with the oil over medium heat, add the sausage and brown for 5 minutes.
2. Add the onion, carrots, garlic and celery and sauté for 3 minutes more.
3. Add the rest of the ingredients except the parmesan, bring to a simmer and cook over medium heat for 30 minutes.
4. Discard the bay leaf, ladle the soup into bowls, sprinkle the parmesan on top and serve.
Nutrition: calories 564, fat 26.5, fiber 15.4, carbs 37.4, protein 26.6

Fish Soup

Preparation time: 10 minutes
Cooking time: 20 minutes
Servings: 4
Ingredients:
- 2 tablespoons olive oil
- 1 tablespoon garlic, minced
- ½ cup tomatoes, crushed
- 1 yellow onion, chopped
- 1 quart veggie stock
- 1 pound cod, skinless, boneless and cubed
- ¼ teaspoon rosemary, dried
- A pinch of salt and black pepper

Directions:
1. Heat up a pot with the oil over medium heat, add the onion and the garlic and sauté for 5 minutes.
2. Add the rest of the ingredients, toss, simmer over medium heat for 15 minutes more, divide into bowls and serve for lunch.

Nutrition: calories 198, fat 8.1, fiber 1, carbs 4.2, protein 26.4

Chickpeas Soup

Preparation time: 10 minutes
Cooking time: 1 hour
Servings: 4
Ingredients:

- 3 tomatoes, cubed
- 2 yellow onions, chopped
- 2 tablespoons olive oil
- 4 celery stalks, chopped
- ½ cup parsley, chopped
- 2 garlic cloves, minced
- 16 ounces canned chickpeas, drained and rinsed
- 6 cups water
- 1 teaspoon cumin, ground
- Juice of ½ lemon
- 1 teaspoon turmeric powder
- ½ teaspoon cinnamon powder
- ½ teaspoon ginger, grated
- Salt and black pepper to the taste

Directions:
1. Heat up a pot with the oil over medium heat, add the onion and the garlic and sauté for 5 minutes.
2. Add the tomatoes, celery, cumin, turmeric, cinnamon and the ginger, stir and sauté for 5 minutes more.
3. Add the remaining ingredients, bring the soup to a boil over medium heat and simmer for 50 minutes.
4. Ladle the soup into bowls and serve.
Nutrition: calories 300, fat 15.4, fiber 4.5, carbs 29.5, protein 15.4

Tomato Soup

Preparation time: 10 minutes
Cooking time: 55 minutes
Servings: 8
Ingredients:

- 4 pounds tomatoes, halved
- 2 tablespoons olive oil
- 6 garlic cloves, minced
- 1 yellow onion, chopped
- Salt and black pepper to the taste
- 4 cups chicken stock
- ½ teaspoon red pepper flakes
- ½ cup basil, chopped
- ½ cup parmesan, grated

Directions:
1. Arrange the tomatoes in a roasting pan, add half of the oil, salt and pepper, toss, and bake at 400 degrees F for 20 minutes.
2. Heat up a pot with the rest of the oil over medium heat, add the onion and sauté for 5 minutes.
3. Add the tomatoes and the rest of the ingredients except the basil and the parmesan, bring to a simmer and cook for 30 minutes.

4. Blend the soup using an immersion blender, add the basil and the parmesan, stir, divide into bowls and serve.
Nutrition: calories 237, fat 10, fiber 3.4, carbs 15.3, protein 7.4

Oyster Stew

Preparation time: 10 minutes
Cooking time: 1 hour and 10 minutes
Servings: 6
Ingredients:

- 2 garlic cloves, minced
- ¼ cup jarred roasted red peppers
- 2 teaspoons oregano, chopped
- 1 pound lamb meat, ground
- 1 tablespoon red wine vinegar
- Salt and black pepper to the taste
- 1 teaspoon red pepper flakes
- 2 tablespoons olive oil
- 1 and ½ cups chicken stock
- 36 oysters, shucked
- 1 and ½ cups canned black eyed peas, drained

Directions:
1. Heat up a pot with the oil over medium heat, add the meat and the garlic and brown for 5 minutes.
2. Add the peppers and the rest of the ingredients, bring to a simmer and cook for 15 minutes.
3. Divide the stew into bowls and serve.
Nutrition: calories 264, fat 9.3, fiber 1.2, carbs 2.3, protein 1.2

Potatoes and Lentils Stew

Preparation time: 10 minutes
Cooking time: 35 minutes
Servings: 4
Ingredients:

4 cups water
- 1 cup carrots, sliced
- 1 yellow onion, chopped
- 1 tablespoon olive oil
- 1 cup celery, chopped
- 2 garlic cloves, minced
- 2 pounds gold potatoes, cubed
- 1 and ½ cup lentils, dried
- ½ teaspoon smoked paprika
- ½ teaspoon oregano, dried
- Salt and black pepper to the taste
- 14 ounces canned tomatoes, chopped
- ½ cup cilantro, chopped

Directions:
1. Heat up a pot with the oil over medium- high heat, add the onion, garlic, celery and carrots, stir and cook for 5 minutes.
2. Add the rest of the ingredients except the cilantro, stir, bring to a simmer and cook over medium heat for 25 minutes.
3. Add the cilantro, divide the stew into bowls and serve.
Nutrition: calories 325, fat 17.3, fiber 6.8, carbs 26.4, protein 16.4

Lamb and Potatoes Stew

Preparation time: 10 minutes
Cooking time: 1 hour and 20 minutes
Servings: 4
Ingredients:
- 2 pounds lamb shoulder, boneless and cubed
- Salt and black pepper to the taste
- 1 yellow onion, chopped
- 3 tablespoons olive oil
- 3 tomatoes, grated
- 2 cups chicken stock
- 2 and ½ pounds gold potatoes, cubed
- ¾ cup green olives, pitted and sliced
- 1 tablespoon cilantro, chopped

Directions:
1. Heat up a pot with the oil over medium-high heat, add the lamb, and brown for 5 minutes on each side.
2. Add the onion and sauté for 5 minutes more.
3. Add the rest of the ingredients, bring to a simmer and cook over medium heat and cook for 1 hour and 10 minutes.
4. Divide the stew into bowls and serve.

Nutrition: calories 411, fat 17.4, fiber 8.4, carbs 25.5, protein 34.3

Ground Pork and Tomatoes Soup

Preparation time: 10 minutes
Cooking time: 40 minutes
Servings: 4
Ingredients:
- 1 pound pork meat, ground
- Salt and black pepper to the taste
- 2 garlic cloves, minced
- 2 teaspoons thyme, dried
- 2 tablespoons olive oil
- 4 cups beef stock
- A pinch of saffron powder
- 15 ounces canned tomatoes, crushed
- 1 tablespoons parsley, chopped

Directions:
1. Heat up a pot with the oil over medium heat, add the meat and the garlic and brown for 5 minutes.
2. Add the rest of the ingredients except the parsley, bring to a simmer and cook for 25 minutes.
3. Divide the soup into bowls, sprinkle the parsley on top and serve.

Nutrition: calories 372, fat 17.3, fiber 5.5, carbs 28.4, protein 17.4

Peas Soup

Preparation time: 10 minutes
Cooking time: 10 minutes
Servings: 4
Ingredients:
- 1 white onion, chopped
- 1 tablespoon olive oil
- 1 quart veggie stock
- 2 eggs
- 3 tablespoons lemon juice
- 2 cups peas
- 2 tablespoons parmesan, grated
- Salt and black pepper to the taste

Directions:
1. Heat up a pot with the oil over medium-high heat, add the onion and sauté for 4 minutes.
2. Add the rest of the ingredients except the eggs, bring to a simmer and cook for 4 minutes.
3. Add whisked eggs, stir the soup, cook for 2 minutes more, divide into bowls and serve.

Nutrition: calories 293, fat 11.2 fiber 3.4, carbs 27, protein 4.45

Minty Lamb Stew

Preparation time: 10 minutes
Cooking time: 1 hour and 45 minutes
Servings: 4
Ingredients:
- 3 cups orange juice
- ½ cup mint, chopped
- Salt and black pepper to the taste
- 2 pounds lamb shoulder, boneless and cubed
- 3 tablespoons olive oil
- 1 carrot, chopped
- 1 yellow onion, chopped
- 1 celery rib, chopped
- 1 tablespoon ginger, grated
- 28 ounces canned tomatoes, crushed
- 1 tablespoon garlic, minced
- 1 cup apricots, dried and halved
- ½ cup mint, chopped
- 15 ounces canned chickpeas, drained
- 6 tablespoons Greek yogurt

Directions:
1. Heat up a pot with 2 tablespoons oil over medium-high heat, add the meat and brown for 5 minutes.
2. Add the carrot, onion, celery, garlic and the ginger, stir and sauté for 5 minutes more.
3. Add the rest of the ingredients except the yogurt, bring to a simmer and cook over medium heat for 1 hour and 30 minutes.
4. Divide the stew into bowls, top each serving with the yogurt and serve.

Nutrition: calories 355, fat 14.3, fiber 6.7, carbs 22.6, protein 15.4

Peas and Orzo Soup

Preparation time: 10 minutes
Cooking time: 10 minutes
Servings: 4
Ingredients:
- ½ cup orzo
- 6 cups chicken soup
- 1 and ½ cups cheddar, shredded
- Salt and black pepper to the taste
- 2 teaspoons oregano, dried
- ¼ cup yellow onion, chopped
- 3 cups baby spinach
- 2 tablespoons lime juice

- ½ cup peas

Directions:

1. Heat up a pot with the soup over medium heat, add the orzo and the rest of the ingredients except the cheese, bring to a simmer and cook for 10 minutes.
2. Add the cheese, stir, divide into bowls and serve.

Nutrition: calories 360, fat 10.2, fiber 4.7, carbs 43.3, protein 22.3

Turmeric Chard Soup

Preparation time: 10 minutes
Cooking time: 40 minutes
Servings: 6
Ingredients:

- 2 tablespoons olive oil
- 1 pound chard, chopped
- 1 teaspoon coriander seeds, ground
- 2 teaspoons mustard seeds
- 2 teaspoons garlic, minced
- 1 tablespoon ginger, grated
- ¼ teaspoon cardamom, ground
- ¼ teaspoon turmeric powder
- 1 yellow onion, chopped
- ¾ cup rhubarb, sliced
- Salt and black pepper to the taste
- 5 cups water
- 3 tablespoons cilantro, chopped
- 6 tablespoons yogurt

Directions:

1. Heat up a pan with the oil over medium heat, add the coriander, mustard seeds, garlic, ginger, cardamom, turmeric and the onion, stir and sauté for 5 minutes.
2. Add the rest of the ingredients except the cilantro and the yogurt, bring to a simmer and cook for 20 minutes.
3. Divide the soup into bowls, top each serving with cilantro and yogurt and serve.

Nutrition: calories 189, fat 8.3, fiber 3.4, carbs 11.7, protein 4.5

Chicken and Onions Stew

Preparation time: 10 minutes
Cooking time: 1 hour
Servings: 4
Ingredients:

- 3 garlic cloves, minced
- 3 tablespoons cilantro, chopped
- Salt and black pepper to the taste
- 1 teaspoon ginger, grated
- 2 cups chicken stock
- 2 tablespoons olive oil
- 3 red onions, thinly sliced
- 2 chicken breasts, skinless, boneless and cubed
- 5 ounces apricots, dried and halved
- 2 tablespoons olive oil
- 2/3 cup walnuts, chopped

Directions:

1. Heat up a pot with the oil over medium heat, add the onions, ginger and the garlic and sauté for 5 minutes.
2. Add the meat and brown for 5 minutes more.
3. Add the rest of the ingredients except the cilantro, bring to a simmer and cook over medium heat for 50 minutes.
4. Add the cilantro, stir, divide the stew into bowls and serve.

Nutrition: calories 309, fat 25.4, fiber 4, carbs 15.3, protein 6.7

Sea Bass and Veggies Stew

Preparation time: 10 minutes
Cooking time: 45 minutes
Servings: 4
Ingredients:

- 2 tablespoons parsley, chopped
- 2 tomatoes, peeled and chopped
- 2 tablespoons cilantro, chopped
- 2 garlic cloves, minced
- ½ teaspoon sweet paprika
- 2 cups chicken stock
- ½ teaspoon cumin, ground
- Salt and black pepper to the taste
- 4 black bass fillets, boneless, skinless and cubed
- ¼ cup olive oil
- 3 carrots, sliced
- 1 red bell pepper, chopped
- 1 and ¼ pounds potatoes, peeled and cubed
- ½ cup black olives, pitted and halved
- 1 red onion, sliced

Directions:

1. Heat up a pot with the oil over medium heat, add the garlic, cumin, carrots, bell pepper, onion and the potatoes, and sauté for 10 minutes.
2. Add the rest of the ingredients except the fish, bring to a simmer and cook over medium heat for 25 minutes.
3. Add the fish, cook the stew for 10 minutes more, divide into bowls and serve.

Nutrition: calories 272, fat 15, fiber 3.6, carbs 14, protein 2.3

Tomato Gazpacho

Preparation time: 1 hour
Cooking time: 0 minutes
Servings: 4
Ingredients:

- ½ green bell pepper, chopped
- ½ red bell pepper, chopped
- 1 and ¾ pounds tomatoes, chopped
- 3 tablespoons olive oil
- 1 garlic clove, minced
- 2 teaspoons balsamic vinegar
- Salt and black pepper to the taste
- 1 tablespoon cilantro, chopped

Directions:

1.   In your blender, the peppers with the tomatoes and the rest of the ingredients except the cilantro, pulse well and divide into bowls.
2.   Sprinkle the cilantro on top and serve really cold.
Nutrition: calories 200, fat 7.8, fiber 3.4, carbs 11.4, protein 8.2

Rosemary Kale Soup
Preparation time: 10 minutes
Cooking time: 25 minutes
Servings: 4
Ingredients:
- 1 pound kale, torn
- Salt and black pepper to the taste
- 3 tablespoons olive oil
- 1 celery stalk, chopped
- 1 yellow onion, chopped
- 1 carrot, chopped
- 14 ounces canned tomatoes, chopped
- 2 tablespoons rosemary, chopped
- 4 cups veggie stock

Directions:
1.   Heat up a pot with the oil over medium heat, add the onion, celery and the carrot and sauté for 5 minutes.
2.   Add the rest of the ingredients, simmer the soup over medium heat for 20 minutes, ladle into bowls and serve.
Nutrition: calories 192, fat 8.3, fiber 4.5, carbs 12.3, protein 4.5

Shrimp and Halibut Stew
Preparation time: 10 minutes
Cooking time: 30 minutes
Servings: 6
Ingredients:
- 2 garlic cloves, minced
- 2 tablespoons olive oil
- 1 yellow onion, chopped
- 14 ounces canned tomatoes, chopped
- 1 tablespoon orange zest, grated
- 4 and ½ cups seafood stock
- 1 pound halibut fillets, boneless, skinless and cubed
- 20 shrimp, peeled and deveined
- 1 bunch parsley, chopped
- Salt and white pepper to the taste

Directions:
1.   Heat up a pot with the oil over medium high heat, add the onion and the garlic and sauté for 5 minutes.
2.   Add the tomatoes, orange zest and the stock, stir, bring to a boil and simmer for 20 minutes over medium heat.
3.   Add the fish and the shrimp, cook for 5 minutes more, divide into bowls, sprinkle the parsley on top and serve.
Nutrition: calories 300, fat 14.3, fiber 4.5, carbs 16.1, protein 11

Chili Watermelon Soup
Preparation time: 4 hours
Cooking time: 0 minutes
Servings: 4
Ingredients:
- 2 pounds watermelon, peeled and cubed
- ½ teaspoon chipotle chili powder
- 2 tablespoons olive oil
- A pinch of salt and white pepper
- 1 tomato, chopped
- 1 shallot, chopped
- ¼ cup cilantro, chopped
- 1 small cucumber, chopped
- 2 tablespoons lemon juice
- ½ tablespoon red wine vinegar

Directions:
1.   In a blender, combine the watermelon with the chili powder, the oil and the rest of the ingredients except the vinegar and the lemon juice, pulse well, and divide into bowls.
2.   Top each serving with lemon juice and vinegar and serve.
Nutrition: calories 120, fat 4.5, fiber 3.4, carbs 12, protein 2.3

Shrimp Soup
Preparation time: 10 minutes
Cooking time: 5 minutes
Servings: 6
Ingredients:
- 1 cucumber, chopped
- 3 cups tomato juice
- 3 roasted red peppers, chopped
- 3 tablespoons olive oil
- 2 tablespoons balsamic vinegar
- 1 garlic clove, minced
- Salt and black pepper to the taste
- ½ teaspoon cumin, ground
- 1 pounds shrimp, peeled and deveined
- 1 teaspoon thyme, chopped

Directions:
1.   In your blender, mix cucumber with tomato juice, red peppers, 2 tablespoons oil, the vinegar, cumin, salt, pepper and the garlic, pulse well, transfer to a bowl and keep in the fridge for 10 minutes.
2.   Heat up a pot with the rest of the oil over medium heat, add the shrimp, salt, pepper and the thyme and cook for 2 minutes on each side.
3.   Divide cold soup into bowls, top with the shrimp and serve.
Nutrition: calories 263, fat 11.1, fiber 2.4, carbs 12.5, protein 6.32

Mussels and Veggies Stew
Preparation time: 10 minutes
Cooking time: 30 minutes
Servings: 4
Ingredients:
- 1 yellow onion, chopped
- 2 tablespoons olive oil

- 1 fennel bulb, chopped
- 1 carrot, chopped
- 1 red bell pepper, chopped
- 2 garlic cloves, minced
- 3 tablespoons tomato paste
- 16 ounces canned chickpeas, drained
- 1 teaspoon thyme, dried
- ¼ teaspoon smoked paprika
- Salt and black pepper to the taste
- 3 and ½ cups water
- 1 pound mussels, scrubbed

Directions:
1.   Heat up a pot with the oil over medium high heat, add the fennel, onion, bell pepper and carrot, stir and cook for 5 minutes.
2.   Add the garlic and tomato paste, stir and cook for 1 minute more.
3.   Add the rest of the ingredients except the mussels, stir, bring to a simmer and cook for 20 minutes.
4.   Add the mussels, cook the stew for 4-5 minutes more, divide into bowls and serve.
Nutrition: calories 450, fat 12, fiber 13, carbs 47, protein 34

Grapes, Cucumbers and Almonds Soup

Preparation time: 10 minutes
Cooking time: 0 minutes
Servings: 4
Ingredients:
- ¼ cup almonds, chopped and toasted
- 3 cucumbers, peeled and chopped
- 3 garlic cloves, minced
- ½ cup warm water
- 6 scallions, sliced
- ¼ cup white wine vinegar
- 3 tablespoons olive oil
- Salt and white pepper to the taste
- 1 teaspoon lemon juice
- ½ cup green grapes, halved

Directions:
1.   In your blender, combine the almonds with the cucumbers and the rest of the ingredients except the grapes and lemon juice, pulse well and divide into bowls.
2.   Top each serving with the lemon juice and grapes and serve cold.
Nutrition: calories 200, fat 5.4, fiber 2.4, carbs 7.6, protein 3.3

Tomato, Sweet Potatoes and Olives Stew

Preparation time: 10 minutes
Cooking time: 30 minutes
Servings: 4
Ingredients:
- 1 yellow onion, chopped
- 1 tablespoon olive oil
- 2 cups sweet potatoes, peeled and chopped
- 1 and ½ teaspoon cumin, ground
- 20 ounces canned tomatoes, chopped
- 1 and ½ teaspoon honey
- 6 tablespoons orange juice
- 1 cup water
- Salt and black pepper to the taste
- ½ cup green olives, pitted and halved
- 1 tablespoon cilantro, chopped

Directions:
1.   Heat up a pot with the oil over medium heat, add the onion, stir and sauté for 5 minutes.
2.   Add the rest of the ingredients, stir, bring to a simmer and cook over medium heat for 25 minutes.
3.   Divide the stew into bowls and serve.
Nutrition: calories 235, fat 12.3, fiber 3.5, carbs 16.3, protein 10.2

Mint Chicken Soup

Preparation time: 10 minutes
Cooking time: 30 minutes
Servings: 4
Ingredients:
- Salt and black pepper to the taste
- 6 cups chicken stock
- ¼ cup lemon juice
- 1 chicken breast, boneless, skinless and cubed
- ½ cup white rice
- 6 tablespoons mint, chopped

Directions:
1.   Put the stock in a pot, add salt and pepper, bring to a simmer over medium heat, add the rice and cook for 15 minutes.
2.   Add the rest of the ingredients, stir, cook for 15 minutes more, divide into bowls and serve.
Nutrition: calories 232, fat 11, fiber 2.4, carbs 14.3, protein 12.4

Spiced Eggplant Stew

Preparation time: 10 minutes
Cooking time: 45 minutes
Servings: 4
Ingredients:
- 4 eggplants, cubed
- Salt and black pepper to the taste
- 2 yellow onions, chopped
- 2 red bell peppers, chopped
- 30 ounces canned tomatoes, chopped
- 1 cup black olives, pitted and chopped
- ¼ teaspoon allspice, ground
- ½ teaspoon cinnamon powder
- 1 teaspoon oregano, dried
- A drizzle of olive oil
- A pinch of red chili flakes
- 3 tablespoons Greek yogurt

Directions:
1.   Heat up a pot with the oil over medium high heat, add the onions, bell pepper, oregano, cinnamon and the allspice and sauté fro 5 minutes.

2.   Add the rest of the ingredients except the flakes and the yogurt, bring to a simmer and cook over medium heat for 40 minutes.
3.   Divide the stew into bowls, top each serving with the flakes and the yogurt and serve.
Nutrition: calories 256, fat 3.5, fiber 25.4, carbs 53.3, protein 8.8

Creamy Salmon Soup

Preparation time: 10 minutes
Cooking time: 15 minutes
Servings: 6
Ingredients:
- 2 tablespoon olive oil
- 1 red onion, chopped
- Salt and white pepper to the taste
- 3 gold potatoes, peeled and cubed
- 2 carrots, chopped
- 4 cups fish stock
- 4 ounces salmon fillets, boneless and cubed
- ½ cup heavy cream
- 1 tablespoon dill, chopped

Directions:
1.   Heat up a pan with the oil over medium heat, add the onion, and sauté for 5 minutes.
2.   Add the rest of the ingredients expect the cream, salmon and the dill, bring to a simmer and cook for 5-6 minutes more.
3.   Add the salmon, cream and the dill, simmer for 5 minutes more, divide into bowls and serve.
Nutrition: calories 214, fat 16.3, fiber 1.5, carbs 6.4, protein 11.8

Chicken and Beans Soup

Preparation time: 10 minutes
Cooking time: 1 hour
Servings: 6
Ingredients:
- 2 tablespoons olive oil
- 2 yellow onions, chopped
- 3 tomatoes, chopped
- 4 cups chicken stock
- 1 pound chicken breasts, skinless, boneless and cubed
- 3 garlic cloves, minced
- 3 red chili peppers, chopped
- 1 tablespoon coriander seeds, crushed
- 14 ounces canned black beans, drained
- Zest of 1 lime, grated
- Juice of 1 lime
- Salt and black pepper to the taste
- 1 tablespoon coriander, chopped

Directions:
1.   Heat up a pot with the oil over medium heat, add the onions, the chicken, garlic, chili peppers and the coriander and sauté for 10 minutes.
2.   Add the rest of the ingredients, bring to a simmer over medium heat, cook for 50 minutes, ladle into bowls and serve.

Nutrition: calories 667, fat 17.6, fiber 17.6, carbs 72.3, protein 55.4

Creamy Chicken Soup

Preparation time: 10 minutes
Cooking time: 1 hour
Servings: 8
Ingredients:
- 2 cups eggplant, cubed
- Salt and black pepper to the taste
- ¼ cup olive oil
- 1 yellow onion, chopped
- 2 tablespoons garlic, minced
- 1 red bell pepper, chopped
- 2 tablespoons hot paprika
- ¼ cup parsley, chopped
- 1 and ½ tablespoons oregano, chopped
- 4 cups chicken stock
- 1 pound chicken breast, skinless, boneless and cubed
- 1 cup half and half
- 2 egg yolks
- ¼ cup lime juice

Directions:
1.   Heat up a pot with the oil over medium heat, add the chicken, garlic and onion, and brown for 10 minutes.
2.   Add the bell pepper and the rest of the ingredients except the half and half, egg, yolks and the lime juice, bring to a simmer and cook over medium heat for 40 minutes.
3.   In a bowl, combine the egg yolks with the remaining ingredients with 1 cup of soup, whisk well and pour into the pot.
4.   Whisk the soup, cook for 5 minutes more, divide into bowls and serve.
Nutrition: calories 312, fat 17.4, fiber 5.6, carbs 20.2, protein 15.3

Chicken, Carrots and Lentils Soup

Preparation time: 10 minutes
Cooking time: 1 hour and 10 minutes
Servings: 8
Ingredients:
- 4 tablespoons olive oil
- 2 carrots, chopped
- 1 yellow onion, chopped
- 2 tablespoons tomato paste
- 2 garlic cloves, chopped
- 6 cups chicken stock
- 2 cups brown lentils, dried
- 1 pound chicken thighs, skinless, boneless and cubed
- Salt and black pepper to the taste

Directions:
1.   Heat up a pot with the oil over medium high heat, add the chicken, onion and the garlic and brown for 10 minutes.
2.   Add the rest of the ingredients, bring the soup to a boil and simmer for 1 hour.

3.   Ladle the soup into bowls and serve for lunch.
Nutrition: calories 311, fat 13.2, fiber 4.3, carbs 17.5, protein 13.4

Pork and Rice Soup

Preparation time: 5 minutes
Cooking time: 7 hours
Servings: 4
Ingredients:

- 2 pounds pork stew meat, cubed
- A pinch of salt and black pepper
- 6 cups water
- 1 leek, sliced
- 2 bay leaves
- 1 carrot, sliced
- 3 tablespoons olive oil
- 1 cup white rice
- 2 cups yellow onion, chopped
- ½ cup lemon juice
- 1 tablespoon cilantro, chopped

Directions:
1.   In your slow cooker, combine the pork with the water and the rest of the ingredients except the cilantro, put the lid on and cook on Low for 7 hours.
2.   Stir the soup, ladle into bowls, sprinkle the cilantro on top and serve.
Nutrition: calories 300, fat 15, fiber 7.6, carbs 17.4, protein 22.4

Barley and Chicken Soup

Preparation time: 10 minutes
Cooking time: 50 minutes
Servings: 6
Ingredients:

- 1 pound chicken breasts, skinless, boneless and cubed
- 1 tablespoon olive oil
- Salt and black pepper to the taste
- 2 celery stalks, chopped
- 2 carrots, chopped
- 1 red onion, chopped
- 6 cups chicken stock
- ½ cup parsley, chopped
- ½ cup barley
- 1 teaspoon lime juice

Directions:
1.   Heat up a pot with the oil over medium high heat, add the chicken, season with salt and pepper, and brown for cook for 8 minutes.
2.   Add the onion, carrots and the celery, stir and cook for 3 minutes more.
3.   Add the rest of the ingredients except the parsley, bring to a boil and simmer over medium heat for 40 minutes.
4.   Add the parsley, stir, divide the soup into bowls and serve.
Nutrition: calories 311, fat 8.4, fiber 8.3, carbs 17.4, protein 22.3

Mushrooms and Chicken Soup

Preparation time: 10 minutes
Cooking time: 30 minutes
Servings: 4
Ingredients:

- 1 red onion, chopped
- 1 tablespoon olive oil
- 2 celery stalks, chopped
- 2 garlic cloves, minced
- 2 carrots chopped
- Salt and black pepper to the taste
- 1 tablespoon thyme, chopped
- 1 qt chicken stock
- 4 ounces white mushrooms, sliced
- 1 cup heavy cream
- 4 cups rotisserie chicken, shredded
- 2 tablespoons cilantro, chopped

Directions:
1.   Heat up a pot with the oil over medium heat, add the onion, celery, garlic, carrot and thyme, and sauté for 5 minutes.
2.   Add the rest of the ingredients except the cream and the cilantro, stir, bring to a boil and cook for 20 minutes.
3.   Add the cream and cilantro, stir, cook the soup for 5 minutes more, divide everything into bowls and serve.
Nutrition: calories 287, fat 11.3, fiber 8.7, carbs 22.4, protein 14.4

Pork and Lentils Soup

Preparation time: 10 minutes
Cooking time: 1 hour
Servings: 6
Ingredients:

- 1 yellow onion, chopped
- 1 tablespoon olive oil
- 2 teaspoons basil, dried
- 1 and ½ teaspoons ginger, grated
- 3 garlic cloves, chopped
- Salt and black pepper to the taste
- 1 carrot, chopped
- 1 pound pork stew meat, cubed
- 3 ounces brown lentils, rinsed
- 4 cups chicken stock
- 2 tablespoons tomato paste
- 2 tablespoons lime juice

Directions:
1.   Heat up a pot with the oil over medium heat, add the meat, onion and the garlic and brown for 6 minutes.
2.   Add the rest of the ingredients, bring the soup to a boil and cook for 55 minutes.
3.   Divide the soup into bowls and serve.
Nutrition: calories 263, fat 11.3, fiber 4.5, carbs 24.4, protein 14.4

Nutmeg Beef Soup

Preparation time: 10 minutes
Cooking time: 30 minutes

Servings: 8
Ingredients:
- 1 yellow onion, chopped
- 1 tablespoon olive oil
- 1 garlic clove, minced
- 1 pound beef meat, ground
- 1 pound eggplant, chopped
- ¾ cup carrots, chopped
- Salt and black pepper to the taste
- 30 ounces canned tomatoes, drained and chopped
- 1 quart beef stock
- ½ teaspoon nutmeg, ground
- 2 teaspoons parsley, chopped

Directions:
1. Heat up a pot with the oil over medium heat, add the meat, onion and the garlic and brown for 5 minutes.
2. Add the rest of the ingredients except the parsley, bring to a boil and cook over medium heat for 25 minutes.
3. Add the parsley, divide the soup into bowls and serve.
Nutrition: calories 232, fat 5.4, fiber 7.6, carbs 20.1, protein 6.5

Herbed Beef and Tomato Soup
Preparation time: 10 minutes
Cooking time: 1 hour
Servings: 8
Ingredients:
- 1 pound beef stew meat, cubed
- 2 tablespoons olive oil
- 2 celery stalks, chopped
- 2 carrots, chopped
- 1 yellow onion, chopped
- Salt and black pepper to the taste
- 3 garlic cloves, chopped
- 1 quart chicken stock
- 1 and ½ teaspoons cilantro, dried
- 1 teaspoon oregano, dried
- 28 ounces canned tomatoes, chopped
- ¼ cup parsley, chopped

Directions:
1. Heat up a pot with the oil over medium high heat, add the meat, onion and the garlic and brown for 10 minutes.
2. Add the rest of the ingredients except the parsley, bring the soup to a boil and simmer for 50 minutes.
3. Add the parsley, divide the soup into bowls and serve.
Nutrition: calories 347, fat 15.2, fiber 4.2, carbs 15.5, protein 37.7

Baked Beef and Onions Stew
Preparation time: 10 minutes
Cooking time: 2 hours and 10 minutes
Servings: 6

Ingredients:
- 2 tablespoons olive oil
- 2 pounds beef meat, cubed
- 1 pound carrots, chopped
- 3 garlic cloves, chopped
- 2 yellow onions, chopped
- 3 cups beef stock
- 2 tablespoons tomato paste
- 1 teaspoon thyme, chopped
- 1 pound pearl onions
- 3 bay leaves
- 1 pound white mushrooms, sliced
- Salt and black pepper to the taste

Directions:
1. Heat up a Dutch oven with the oil over medium heat, add the meat, salt and pepper and brown for 5 minutes.
2. Add the onions and the garlic and brown for 5 minutes more.
3. Add the rest of the ingredients, introduce the pot in the oven and bake at 350 degrees F for 2 hours.
4. Divide the stew into bowls and serve.
Nutrition: calories 221, fat 8, fiber 8, carbs 33.1, protein 8.9

Beef and Cucumber Mix
Preparation time: 10 minutes
Cooking time: 10 minutes
Servings: 4
Ingredients:
- 1 pound beef steaks, sliced
- 4 cucumbers, cut with a spiralizer
- ½ cup sweet chili sauce
- 1 cup carrot, grated
- ½ cup water
- 1 tablespoon olive oil
- 1 tablespoon chives, chopped
- Salt and black pepper to the taste

Directions:
1. Heat up a pan with the oil over medium-high heat, add the steaks, and cook for 4 minutes on each side.
2. Add the cucumber noodles and the rest of the ingredients, cook for 2 minutes more, divide between plates and serve.
Nutrition: calories 357, fat 10.9, fiber 2.2, carbs 25.7, protein 36.6

Parsley Beef Stew
Preparation time: 10 minutes
Cooking time: 7 hours
Servings: 4
Ingredients:
- 2 pounds beef stew meat, cubed
- Salt and black pepper to the taste
- 2 cups beef stock
- 2 tablespoons olive oil
- 1 yellow onion, chopped
- 2 tablespoons thyme, chopped
- 4 garlic cloves, minced

- 3 carrots, chopped
- 3 celery stalks, chopped
- 28 ounces canned tomatoes, crushed
- ½ cup parsley, chopped

Directions:

1. In your slow cooker, combine the beef with the stock and all the other ingredients, put the lid on and cook on Low for 7 hours.
2. Divide the stew into bowls and serve.

Nutrition: calories 364, fat 16.5, fiber 4.5, carbs 27.6, protein 33.3

Hot Lamb and Carrots Stew

Preparation time: 10 minutes
Cooking time: 8 hours and 10 minutes
Servings: 6
Ingredients:

- 2 carrots, sliced
- 1 tablespoon chili powder
- 1 pound lamb meat, boneless and cubed
- 1 tablespoon olive oil
- Salt and black pepper to the taste
- 2 yellow onions, chopped
- 2 teaspoon peppercorns, crushed
- A pinch of whole allspice
- 3 cups beef stock
- 1 tablespoon dill, chopped

Directions:

1. Heat up a pan with the oil over medium high heat, add the meat, brown for 5 minutes on each side and transfer to the slow cooker.
2. Add the rest of the ingredients except the dill, put the lid on and cook on Low for 8 hours.
3. Divide the stew into bowls and serve with the dill sprinkled on top.

Nutrition: calories 384, fat 23.3, fiber 7.6, carbs 27.8, protein 36.4

Lamb and Artichokes Stew

Preparation time: 10 minutes
Cooking time: 8 hours and 10 minutes
Servings: 8
Ingredients:

- 3 pounds lamb shoulder, boneless and trimmed
- 2 yellow onions, chopped
- 1 tablespoon olive oil
- 1 tablespoon oregano, dried
- 3 garlic cloves, minced
- Salt and black pepper to the taste
- 2 cups beef stock
- 6 ounces canned artichoke hearts, drained
- ¼ cup tomato paste
- ½ cup feta cheese, crumbled
- 2 tablespoons parsley, chopped

Directions:

1. Heat up a pan with the olive oil over medium high heat, add the meat, brown for 10 minutes and transfer to your slow cooker.

2. Add the onions, oregano and the rest of the ingredients except the cheese and the parsley, stir, put the lid on and cook on Low for 8 hours.
3. Divide the stew into bowls, sprinkle the cheese and the parsley on top and serve.

Nutrition: calories 364, fat 18.5, fiber 8.5, carbs 28.7, protein 33.4

Caraway Pork Stew

Preparation time: 10 minutes
Cooking time: 40 minutes
Servings: 6
Ingredients:

- 2 pounds pork stew meat, boneless and cubed
- 2 yellow onions, chopped
- 1 tablespoon olive oil
- 1 garlic clove, minced
- 3 cups beef stock
- 2 tablespoons sweet paprika
- 1 teaspoon caraway seeds, crushed
- Salt and black pepper to the taste
- 2 tablespoons dill, chopped

Directions:

1. Heat up a pot with the oil over medium heat, add the meat brown it for 5 minutes.
2. Add the onions and the garlic and sauté for 5 minutes more.
3. Add the rest of the ingredients, bring the stew to a boil and cook for 30 minutes.
4. Divide the stew into bowls and serve.

Nutrition: calories 322, fat 17.4, fiber 7.6, carbs 26.4, protein 34.3

Coriander Pork and Chickpeas Stew

Preparation time: 10 minutes
Cooking time: 8 hours
Servings: 4
Ingredients:

- ½ cup beef stock
- 1 tablespoon ginger, grated
- 1 teaspoon coriander, ground
- 2 teaspoons cumin, ground
- Salt and black pepper to the taste
- 2 and ½ pounds pork stew meat, cubed
- 28 ounces canned tomatoes, drained and chopped
- 1 red onion, chopped
- 4 garlic cloves, minced
- ½ cup apricots, cut into quarters
- 15 ounces canned chickpeas, drained
- 1 tablespoon cilantro, chopped

Directions:

1. In your slow cooker, combine the meat with the stock, ginger and the rest of the ingredients except the cilantro and the chickpeas, put the lid on and cook on Low for 7 hours and 40 minutes.
2. Add the cilantro and the chickpeas, cook the stew on Low for 20 minutes more, divide into bowls and serve.

Nutrition: calories 283, fat 11.9, fiber 4.5, carbs 28.8, protein 25.4

Sage Pork and Beans Stew
Preparation time: 10 minutes
Cooking time: 4 hours and 10 minutes
Servings: 4
Ingredients:
- 2 pounds pork stew meat, cubed
- 2 tablespoons olive oil
- 1 sweet onion, chopped
- 1 red bell pepper, chopped
- 3 garlic cloves, minced
- 2 teaspoons sage, dried
- 4 ounces canned white beans, drained
- 1 cup beef stock
- 2 zucchinis, chopped
- 2 tablespoons tomato paste
- 1 tablespoon cilantro, chopped

Directions:
1. Heat up a pan with the oil over medium-high heat, add the meat, brown for 10 minutes and transfer to your slow cooker.
2. Add the rest of the ingredients except the cilantro, put the lid on and cook on High for 4 hours.
3. Divide the stew into bowls, sprinkle the cilantro on top and serve.
Nutrition: calories 423, fat 15.4, fiber 9.6, carbs 27.4, protein 43

Bread and Veggies Salad
Preparation time: 10 minutes
Cooking time: 5 minutes
Servings: 6
Ingredients:
- 3 tablespoons olive oil
- 2 pita breads, broken into pieces
- 1 cucumber, sliced
- 1 cup baby arugula
- 3 medium tomatoes, chopped
- 5 green bell peppers, chopped
- 1 cup parsley, chopped
- 5 radishes, sliced

For the dressing:
- 1/3 cup olive oil
- Juice of 1 lime
- Salt and black pepper to the taste
- ½ teaspoon cinnamon powder
- ¼ teaspoon allspice, ground

Directions:
1. Heat up a pan with 3 tablespoons olive oil over medium heat, add the pita pieces, salt and pepper and brown for 5 minutes.
2. In a salad bowl, mix the pita with the cucumber, arugula, tomatoes, bell pepper, parsley and the radishes and toss.
3. In a separate bowl, combine 1/3 cup oil with the rest of the ingredients for the dressing, whisk well, pour over the salad, toss and serve for lunch.

Nutrition: calories 277, fat 7.8, fiber 4.5, carbs 26, protein 11.2

Potato Soup
Preparation time: 10 minutes
Cooking time: 30 minutes
Servings: 2
Ingredients:
- 2 medium potatoes, peeled and cubed
- 1 white onion, chopped
- 2 tablespoons olive oil
- 1 small carrot, cubed
- 3 cups chicken stock
- Salt and black pepper to the taste
- 1 tablespoon chives, chopped
- 1 tablespoon cilantro, chopped

Directions:
1. Heat up a pot with the oil over medium heat, add the onion and the carrot and cook for 5 minutes.
2. Add the potatoes and sauté for 5 more minutes.
3. Add the stock, salt and pepper, bring to a simmer and cook over medium heat for 20 minutes.
4. Add the chives and the cilantro, stir, divide the soup into bowls and serve.
Nutrition: calories 245, fat 11.2, fiber 4.5, carbs 17.4, protein 12.3

Side Dish Recipes

Balsamic Asparagus

Preparation time: 10 minutes
Cooking time: 15 minutes
Servings: 4
Ingredients:
- 3 tablespoons olive oil
- 3 garlic cloves, minced
- 2 tablespoons shallot, chopped
- Salt and black pepper to the taste
- 2 teaspoons balsamic vinegar
- 1 and ½ pound asparagus, trimmed

Directions:
1. Heat up a pan with the oil over medium-high heat, add the garlic and the shallot and sauté for 3 minutes.
2. Add the rest of the ingredients, cook for 12 minutes more, divide between plates and serve as a side dish.

Nutrition: calories 100, fat 10.5, fiber 1.2, carbs 2.3, protein 2.1

Lime Cucumber Mix

Preparation time: 10 minutes
Cooking time: 0 minutes
Servings: 8
Ingredients:
- 4 cucumbers, chopped
- ½ cup green bell pepper, chopped
- 1 yellow onion, chopped
- 1 chili pepper, chopped
- 1 garlic clove, minced
- 1 teaspoon parsley, chopped
- 2 tablespoons lime juice
- 1 tablespoon dill, chopped
- Salt and black pepper to the taste
- 1 tablespoon olive oil

Directions:
1. In a large bowl, mix the cucumber with the bell peppers and the rest of the ingredients, toss and serve as a side dish.

Nutrition: calories 123, fat 4.3, fiber 2.3, carbs 5.6, protein 2

Walnuts Cucumber Mix

Preparation time: 5 minutes
Cooking time: 0 minutes
Servings: 2
Ingredients:
- 2 cucumbers, chopped
- 1 tablespoon olive oil
- Salt and black pepper to the taste
- 1 red chili pepper, dried
- 1 tablespoon lemon juice
- 3 tablespoons walnuts, chopped
- 1 tablespoon balsamic vinegar
- 1 teaspoon chives, chopped

Directions:

1. In a bowl, mix the cucumbers with the oil and the rest of the ingredients, toss and serve as a side dish.

Nutrition: calories 121, fat 2.3, fiber 2.0, carbs 6.7, protein 2.4

Cheesy Beet Salad

Preparation time: 10 minutes
Cooking time: 1 hour
Servings: 4
Ingredients:
- 4 beets, peeled and cut into wedges
- 3 tablespoons olive oil
- Salt and black pepper to the taste
- ¼ cup lime juice
- 8 slices goat cheese, crumbled
- 1/3 cup walnuts, chopped
- 1 tablespoons chives, chopped

Directions:
1. In a roasting pan, combine the beets with the oil, salt and pepper, toss and bake at 400 degrees F for 1 hour.
2. Cool the beets down, transfer them to a bowl, add the rest of the ingredients, toss and serve as a side salad.

Nutrition: calories 156, fat 4.2, fiber 3.4, carbs 6.5, protein 4

Rosemary Beets

Preparation time: 10 minutes
Cooking time: 20 minutes
Servings: 4
Ingredients:
- 4 medium beets, peeled and cubed
- 1/3 cup balsamic vinegar
- 1 teaspoon rosemary, chopped
- 1 garlic clove, minced
- ½ teaspoon Italian seasoning
- 1 tablespoon olive oil

Directions:
1. Heat up a pan with the oil over medium heat, add the beets and the rest of the ingredients, toss, and cook for 20 minutes.
2. Divide the mix between plates and serve as a side dish.

Nutrition: calories 165, fat 3.4, fiber 4.5, carbs 11.3, protein 2.3

Squash and Tomatoes Mix

Preparation time: 10 minutes
Cooking time: 20 minutes
Servings: 6
Ingredients:
- 5 medium squash, cubed
- A pinch of salt and black pepper
- 3 tablespoons olive oil
- 1 cup pine nuts, toasted
- ¼ cup goat cheese, crumbled
- 6 tomatoes, cubed
- ½ yellow onion, chopped

- 2 tablespoons cilantro, chopped
- 2 tablespoons lemon juice

Directions:
1.   Heat up a pan with the oil over medium heat, add the onion and pine nuts and cook for 3 minutes.
2.   Add the squash and the rest of the ingredients, cook everything for 15 minutes, divide between plates and serve as a side dish.
Nutrition: calories 200, fat 4.5, fiber 3.4, carbs 6.7, protein 4

Balsamic Eggplant Mix

Preparation time: 10 minutes
Cooking time: 20 minutes
Servings: 6
Ingredients:
- 1/3 cup chicken stock
- 2 tablespoons balsamic vinegar
- A pinch of salt and black pepper
- 1 tablespoon lime juice
- 2 big eggplants, sliced
- 1 tablespoon rosemary, chopped
- ¼ cup cilantro, chopped
- 2 tablespoons olive oil

Directions:
1.   In a roasting pan, combine the eggplants with the stock, the vinegar and the rest of the ingredients, introduce the pan in the oven and bake at 390 degrees F for 20 minutes.
2.   Divide the mix between plates and serve as a side dish.
Nutrition: calories 201, fat 4.5, fiber 3, carbs 5.4, protein 3

Sage Barley Mix

Preparation time: 10 minutes
Cooking time: 45 minutes
Servings: 4
Ingredients:
- 1 tablespoon olive oil
- 1 red onion, chopped
- 1 tablespoon leaves, chopped
- 1 garlic clove, minced
- 14 ounces barley
- ½ tablespoon parmesan, grated
- 6 cups veggie stock
- Salt and black pepper to the taste

Directions:
1.   Heat up a pan with the oil over medium heat, add the onion and garlic, stir and sauté for 5 minutes.
2.   Add the sage, barley and the rest of the ingredients except the parmesan, stir, bring to a simmer and cook for 40 minutes,
3.   Add the parmesan, stir, divide between plates.
Nutrition: calories 210, fat 6.5, fiber 3.4, carbs 8.6, protein 3.4

Chickpeas and Beets Mix

Preparation time: 10 minutes
Cooking time: 25 minutes

Servings: 4
Ingredients:
- 3 tablespoons capers, drained and chopped
- Juice of 1 lemon
- Zest of 1 lemon, grated
- 1 red onion, chopped
- 3 tablespoons olive oil
- 14 ounces canned chickpeas, drained
- 8 ounces beets, peeled and cubed
- 1 tablespoon parsley, chopped
- Salt and pepper to the taste

Directions:
1.   Heat up a pan with the oil over medium heat, add the onion, lemon zest, lemon juice and the capers and sauté fro 5 minutes.
2.   Add the rest of the ingredients, stir and cook over medium-low heat for 20 minutes more.
3.   Divide the mix between plates and serve as a side dish.
Nutrition: calories 199, fat 4.5, fiber 2.3, carbs 6.5, protein 3.3

Creamy Sweet Potatoes Mix

Preparation time: 10 minutes
Cooking time: 1 hour
Servings: 4
Ingredients:
- 4 tablespoons olive oil
- 1 garlic clove, minced
- 4 medium sweet potatoes, pricked with a fork
- 1 red onion, sliced
- 3 ounces baby spinach
- Zest and juice of 1 lemon
- A small bunch dill, chopped
- 1 and ½ tablespoons Greek yogurt
- 2 tablespoons tahini paste
- Salt and black pepper to the taste

Directions:
1.   Put the potatoes on a baking sheet lined with parchment paper, introduce in the oven at 350 degrees F and cook them for 1 hour.
2.   Peel the potatoes, cut them into wedges and put them in a bowl.
3.   Add the garlic, the oil and the rest of the ingredients, toss, divide the mix between plates and serve.
Nutrition: calories 214, fat 5.6, fiber 3.4, carbs 6.5, protein 3.1

Cabbage and Mushrooms Mix

Preparation time: 10 minutes
Cooking time: 15 minutes
Servings: 2
Ingredients:
- 1 yellow onion, sliced
- 2 tablespoons olive oil
- 1 tablespoon balsamic vinegar
- ½ pound white mushrooms, sliced
- 1 green cabbage head, shredded
- 4 spring onions, chopped

- Salt and black pepper to the taste

Directions:

1. Heat up a pan with the oil over medium heat, add the yellow onion and the spring onions and cook for 5 minutes.
2. Add the rest of the ingredients, cook everything for 10 minutes, divide between plates and serve.

Nutrition: calories 199, fat 4.5, fiber 2.4, carbs 5.6, protein 2.2

Lemon Mushroom Rice

Preparation time: 10 minutes
Cooking time: 30 minutes
Servings: 4
Ingredients:

- 2 cups chicken stock
- 1 yellow onion, chopped
- ½ pound white mushrooms, sliced
- 2 garlic cloves, minced
- 8 ounces wild rice
- Juice and zest of 1 lemon
- 1 tablespoon chives, chopped
- 6 tablespoons goat cheese, crumbled
- Salt and black pepper to the taste

Directions:

1. Heat up a pot with the stock over medium heat, add the rice, onion and the rest of the ingredients except the chives and the cheese, bring to a simmer and cook for 25 minutes.
2. Add the remaining ingredients, cook everything for 5 minutes, divide between plates and serve as a side dish.

Nutrition: calories 222, fat 5.5, fiber 5.4, carbs 12.3, protein 5.6

Paprika and Chives Potatoes

Preparation time: 10 minutes
Cooking time: 1 hour and 8 minutes
Servings: 4
Ingredients:

- 4 potatoes, scrubbed and pricked with a fork
- 1 tablespoon olive oil
- 1 celery stalk, chopped
- 2 tomatoes, chopped
- 1 teaspoon sweet paprika
- Salt and black pepper to the taste
- 2 tablespoons chives, chopped

Directions:

1. Arrange the potatoes on a baking sheet lined with parchment paper, introduce in the oven and bake at 350 degrees F for 1 hour.
2. Cool the potatoes down, peel and cut them into larger cubes.
3. Heat up a pan with the oil over medium heat, add the celery and the tomatoes and sauté for 2 minutes.
4. Add the potatoes and the rest of the ingredients, toss, cook everything for 6 minutes, divide the mix between plates and serve as a side dish.

Nutrition: calories 233, fat 8.7, fiber 4.5, carbs 14.4, protein 6.4

Bulgur, Kale and Cheese Mix

Preparation time: 10 minutes
Cooking time: 10 minutes
Servings: 6
Ingredients:

- 4 ounces bulgur
- 4 ounces kale, chopped
- 1 tablespoon mint, chopped
- 3 spring onions, chopped
- 1 cucumber, chopped
- A pinch of allspice, ground
- 2 tablespoons olive oil
- Zest and juice of ½ lemon
- 4 ounces feta cheese, crumbled

Directions:

1. Put bulgur in a bowl, cover with hot water, aside for 10 minutes and fluff with a fork.
2. Heat up a pan with the oil over medium heat, add the onions and the allspice and cook for 3 minutes.
3. Add the bulgur and the rest of the ingredients, cook everything for 5-6 minutes more, divide between plates and serve.

Nutrition: calories 200, fat 6.7, fiber 3.4, carbs 15.4, protein 4.5

Spicy Green Beans Mix

Preparation time: 5 minutes
Cooking time: 15 minutes
Servings: 4
Ingredients:

- 4 teaspoons olive oil
- 1 garlic clove, minced
- ½ teaspoon hot paprika
- ¾ cup veggie stock
- 1 yellow onion, sliced
- 1 pound green beans, trimmed and halved
- ½ cup goat cheese, shredded
- 2 teaspoon balsamic vinegar

Directions:

1. Heat up a pan with the oil over medium heat, add the garlic, stir and cook for 1 minute.
2. Add the green beans and the rest of the ingredients, toss, cook everything for 15 minutes more, divide between plates and serve as a side dish.

Nutrition: calories 188, fat 4, fiber 3, carbs 12.4, protein 4.4

Beans and Rice

Preparation time: 10 minutes
Cooking time: 55 minutes
Servings: 6
Ingredients:

- 1 tablespoon olive oil
- 1 yellow onion, chopped
- 2 celery stalks, chopped
- 2 garlic cloves, minced

- 2 cups brown rice
- 1 and ½ cup canned black beans, rinsed and drained
- 4 cups water
- Salt and black pepper to the taste

Directions:
1. Heat up a pan with the oil over medium heat, add the celery, garlic and the onion, stir and cook for 10 minutes.
2. Add the rest of the ingredients, stir, bring to a simmer and cook over medium heat for 45 minutes.
3. Divide between plates and serve.

Nutrition: calories 224, fat 8.4, fiber 3.4, carbs 15.3, protein 6.2

Tomato and Millet Mix

Preparation time: 10 minutes
Cooking time: 20 minutes
Servings: 6
Ingredients:
- 3 tablespoons olive oil
- 1 cup millet
- 2 spring onions, chopped
- 2 tomatoes, chopped
- ½ cup cilantro, chopped
- 1 teaspoon chili paste
- 6 cups cold water
- ½ cup lemon juice
- Salt and black pepper to the taste

Directions:
1. Heat up a pan with the oil over medium heat, add the millet, stir and cook for 4 minutes.
2. Add the water, salt and pepper, stir, bring to a simmer over medium heat cook for 15 minutes.
3. Add the rest of the ingredients, toss, divide the mix between plates and serve as a side dish.

Nutrition: calories 222, fat 10.2, fiber 3.4, carbs 14.5, protein 2.4

Quinoa and Greens Salad

Preparation time: 10 minutes
Cooking time: 0 minutes
Servings: 4
Ingredients:
- 1 cup quinoa, cooked
- 1 medium bunch collard greens, chopped
- 4 tablespoons walnuts, chopped
- 2 tablespoons balsamic vinegar
- 4 tablespoons tahini paste
- 4 tablespoons cold water
- A pinch of salt and black pepper
- 1 tablespoon olive oil

Directions:
1. In a bowl, mix the tahini with the water and vinegar and whisk.
2. In a bowl, mix the quinoa with the rest of the ingredients and the tahini dressing, toss, divide the mix between plates and serve as a side dish.

Nutrition: calories 175, fat 3, fiber 3, carbs 5, protein 3

Veggies and Avocado Dressing

Preparation time: 10 minutes
Cooking time: 0 minutes
Servings: 4
Ingredients:
- 3 tablespoons pepitas, roasted
- 3 cups water
- 2 tablespoons cilantro, chopped
- 4 tablespoons parsley, chopped
- 1 and ½ cups corn
- 1 cup radish, sliced
- 2 avocados, peeled, pitted and chopped
- 2 mangos, peeled and chopped
- 3 tablespoons olive oil
- 4 tablespoons Greek yogurt
- 1 teaspoons balsamic vinegar
- 2 tablespoons lime juice
- Salt and black pepper to the taste

Directions:
1. In your blender, mix the olive oil with avocados, salt, pepper, lime juice, the yogurt and the vinegar and pulse.
2. In a bowl, mix the pepitas with the cilantro, parsley and the rest of the ingredients, and toss.
3. Add the avocado dressing, toss, divide the mix between plates and serve as a side dish.

Nutrition: calories 403, fat 30.5, fiber 10, carbs 23.5, protein 3.5

Dill Beets Salad

Preparation time: 10 minutes
Cooking time: 0 minutes
Servings: 6
Ingredients:
- 2 pounds beets, cooked, peeled and cubed
- 2 tablespoons olive oil
- 1 tablespoon lemon juice
- 2 tablespoons balsamic vinegar
- 1 cup feta cheese, crumbled
- 3 small garlic cloves, minced
- 4 green onions, chopped
- 5 tablespoons parsley, chopped
- Salt and black pepper to the taste

Directions:
1. In a bowl, mix the beets with the oil, lemon juice and the rest of the ingredients, toss and serve as a side dish.

Nutrition: calories 268, fat 15.5, fiber 5.1, carbs 25.7, protein 9.6

Pesto Broccoli Quinoa

Preparation time: 10 minutes
Cooking time: 30 minutes
Servings: 4
Ingredients:
- 2 and ½ cups quinoa
- 4 and ½ cups veggie stock

- A pinch of salt and black pepper
- 2 tablespoons basil pesto
- 2 cups mozzarella cheese, shredded
- 1 pound broccoli florets
- 1/3 cup parmesan, grated
- 2 green onions, chopped

Directions:
1. In a baking pan, combine the quinoa with the stock, and the rest of the ingredients except the parmesan and the mozzarella and toss.
2. Sprinkle the cheese on top and bake everything at 400 degrees F and bake for 30 minutes.
3. Divide between plates and serve as a side dish.

Nutrition: calories 181, fat 3.4, fiber 3.2, carbs 8.6, protein 7.6

Cheesy Peas Mix

Preparation time: 5 minutes
Cooking time: 0 minutes
Servings: 8
Ingredients:
- 2 pounds peas, steamed
- 1 yellow bell pepper, chopped
- 2 ounces feta cheese, grated
- 3 tablespoon basil, chopped
- 1 red onion, chopped
- 1 chili pepper, chopped
- 1 teaspoon apple cider vinegar
- Salt and black pepper to the taste
- 1 tablespoon chives, chopped

Directions:
1. In a salad bowl, mix the peas with the bell pepper and the rest of the ingredients, toss and serve as a side dish.

Nutrition: calories 273, fat 11, fiber 3.4, carbs 7.6, protein 4.9

Cheesy Potato Mash

Preparation time: 10 minutes
Cooking time: 20 minutes
Servings: 8
Ingredients:
- 2 pounds gold potatoes, peeled and cubed
- 1 and ½ cup cream cheese, soft
- Sea salt and black pepper to the taste
- ½ cup almond milk
- 2 tablespoons chives, chopped

Directions:
1. Put potatoes in a pot, add water to cover, add a pinch of salt, bring to a simmer over medium heat, cook for 20 minutes, drain and mash them.
2. Add the rest of the ingredients except the chives and whisk well.
3. Add the chives, stir, divide between plates and serve as a side dish.

Nutrition: calories 243, fat 14.2, fiber 1.4, carbs 3.5, protein 1.4

Rice, Peppers and Onions Mix

Preparation time: 5 minutes

Cooking time: 20 minutes
Servings: 4
Ingredients:
- 2 cups yellow onion, sliced
- 2 cups red bell pepper, cut into strips
- 4 teaspoons olive oil
- 1 cup celery, roughly chopped
- 1 tablespoon garlic, minced
- ¾ cup veggie stock
- ½ cup brown rice
- 1 and ½ cups water
- Salt and black pepper to the taste
- ½ teaspoon thyme, chopped
- ¾ teaspoon sweet paprika
- 4 teaspoons green onions, chopped

Directions:
1. Heat up a pan with the oil over medium-high heat, add the onion, garlic, celery and bell pepper, stir and cook for 10 minutes.
2. Add the rice and the rest of the ingredients, toss, bring to a simmer and cook for 12 minutes.
3. Divide between plates and serve as a side dish.

Nutrition: calories 312, fat 4.5, fiber 8.4, carbs 22.4, protein 4.5

Lemony Barley and Yogurt

Preparation time: 10 minutes
Cooking time: 30 minutes
Servings: 4
Ingredients:
- ½ cup barley
- 1 and ½ cup veggie stock
- ½ cup Greek yogurt
- Salt and black pepper to the taste
- 2 tablespoons olive oil
- 1 tablespoon lemon juice
- ¼ cup mint, chopped
- 1 apple, cored and chopped

Directions:
1. Put barley in a pot, add the stock and salt, bring to a boil and simmer for 30 minutes.
2. Drain, transfer the barley to a bowl, add the rest of the ingredients, toss, divide between plates and serve as a side dish.

Nutrition: calories 263, fat 9, fiber 11.4, carbs 17.4, protein 6.5

Chard and Couscous

Preparation time: 10 minutes
Cooking time: 10 minutes
Servings: 4
Ingredients:
- 10 ounces couscous
- 1 and ½ cup hot water
- 2 garlic cloves, minced
- 2 tablespoons olive oil
- ½ cup raisins
- 2 bunches Swiss chard, chopped
- Salt and black pepper to the taste

Directions:

1. Put couscous in a bowl, add the water, stir, cover, leave aside for 10 minutes and fluff with a fork.
2. Heat up a pan with the oil over medium heat, add the garlic, and sauté for 1 minute.
3. Add the couscous and the rest of the ingredients, toss, divide between plates and serve.
Nutrition: calories 300, fat 6.9, fiber 11.4, carbs 17.4, protein 6

Chili Cabbage and Coconut

Preparation time: 5 minutes
Cooking time: 20 minutes
Servings: 4
Ingredients:
- 3 tablespoons olive oil
- 1 spring curry leaves, chopped
- 1 teaspoon mustard seeds, crushed
- 1 green cabbage head, shredded
- 4 green chili peppers, chopped
- ½ cup coconut flesh, grated
- Salt and black pepper to the taste

Directions:
1. Heat up a pan with the oil over medium heat, add the curry leaves, mustard seeds and the chili peppers and cook for 5 minutes.
2. Add the rest of the ingredients, toss and cook for 15 minutes more.
3. Divide the mix between plates and serve as a side dish.
Nutrition: calories 221, fat 5.5, fiber 11.1, carbs 22.1, protein 6.7

Chickpeas, Figs and Couscous

Preparation time: 10 minutes
Cooking time: 20 minutes
Servings: 4
Ingredients:
- 1 red onion, chopped
- 2 tablespoons olive oil
- 2 garlic cloves, minced
- 28 ounces canned chickpeas, drained and rinsed
- 2 cups veggie stock
- 2 cups couscous, cooked
- 2 tablespoons coriander, chopped
- ½ cup figs, dried and chopped
- Salt and black pepper to the taste

Directions:
1. Heat up a pan with the oil over medium heat, add the onion and the garlic, stir and sauté for 5 minutes.
2. Add the chickpeas and the rest of the ingredients except the couscous and cook over medium heat for 15 minutes stirring often.
3. Divide the couscous between plates, divide the chickpeas mix on top and serve.
Nutrition: calories 263, fat 11.5, fiber 9.45, carbs 22.4, protein 7.3

Cheesy Tomato Salad

Preparation time: 5 minutes

Cooking time: 0 minutes
Servings: 4
Ingredients:
- 2 pounds tomatoes, sliced
- 1 red onion, chopped
- Sea salt and black pepper to the taste
- 4 ounces feta cheese, crumbled
- 2 tablespoons mint, chopped
- A drizzle of olive oil

Directions:
1. In a salad bowl, mix the tomatoes with the onion and the rest of the ingredients, toss and serve as a side salad.
Nutrition: calories 190, fat 4.5, fiber 3.4, carbs 8.7, protein 3.3

Balsamic Tomato Mix

Preparation time: 6 minutes
Cooking time: 0 minutes
Servings: 4
Ingredients:
- 2 pounds cherry tomatoes, halved
- 2 tablespoons olive oil
- 2 tablespoons balsamic vinegar
- 1 garlic clove, minced
- 1 cup basil, chopped
- 1 tablespoon chives, chopped
- Salt and black pepper to the taste

Directions:
1. In a bowl, combine the tomatoes with the garlic, basil and the rest of the ingredients, toss and serve as a side salad.
Nutrition: calories 200, fat 5.6, fiber 4.5, carbs 15.1, protein 4.3

Vinegar Cucumber Mix

Preparation time: 5 minutes
Cooking time: 0 minutes
Servings: 6
Ingredients:
- 1 tablespoon olive oil
- 4 cucumbers, sliced
- Salt and black pepper to the taste
- 1 red onion, chopped
- 3 tablespoons red wine vinegar
- 1 bunch basil, chopped
- 1 teaspoon honey

Directions:
1. In a bowl, mix the vinegar with the basil, salt, pepper, the oil and the honey and whisk well.
2. In a bowl, mix the cucumber with the onion and the vinaigrette, toss and serve as a side salad.
Nutrition: calories 182, fat 7.8, fiber 2.1, carbs 4.3, protein 4.1

Avocado and Onion Mix

Preparation time: 10 minutes
Cooking time: 0 minutes
Servings: 4
Ingredients:

- 4 avocados, pitted, peeled and sliced
- 1 red onion, sliced
- 2 tablespoons olive oil
- 2 tablespoons lime juice
- ¼ cup dill, chopped
- Sea salt and black pepper to the taste

Directions:
1. In a salad bowl, mix the avocados with the onion and the rest of the ingredients, toss and serve as a side dish.

Nutrition: calories 465, fat 23.5, fiber 14.3, carbs 21.4, protein 5.4

Eggplant and Bell Pepper Mix

Preparation time: 10 minutes
Cooking time: 45 minutes
Servings: 4
Ingredients:
- 2 green bell peppers, cut into strips
- 2 eggplants, sliced
- 2 tablespoons tomato paste
- Salt and black pepper to the taste
- 4 garlic cloves, minced
- ¼ cup olive oil
- 1 tablespoon cilantro, chopped
- 1 tablespoon chives, chopped

Directions:
1. In a roasting pan, combine the bell peppers with the eggplants and the rest of the ingredients, introduce in the oven and cook at 380 degrees F for 45 minutes.
2. Divide the mix between plates and serve as a side dish.

Nutrition: calories 207, fat 13.3, fiber 10.5, carbs 23.4, protein 3.8

Basil and Sun-dried Tomatoes Rice

Preparation time: 10 minutes
Cooking time: 25 minutes
Servings: 4
Ingredients:
- 5 cups chicken stock
- 1 yellow onion, chopped
- 10 ounces sun dried tomatoes in olive oil, drained and chopped
- 2 cups Arborio rice
- Salt and black pepper to the taste
- 1 and ½ cup parmesan, grated
- 2 tablespoons olive oil
- ¼ cup basil leaves, chopped

Directions:
1. Heat up a pan with the oil over medium heat, add the onion and the tomatoes and sauté for 5 minutes.
2. Add the rice, stock and the rest of the ingredients except the parmesan, bring to a simmer and cook over medium heat for 20 minutes.
3. Add the parmesan, toss, divide the mix between plates and serve as a side dish.

Nutrition: calories 426, fat 8.4, fiber 3.2, carbs 56.3, protein 7.5

Dill Cucumber Salad

Preparation time: 1 hour
Cooking time: 0 minutes
Servings: 8
Ingredients:
- 4 cucumbers, sliced
- 1 cup white wine vinegar
- 2 white onions, sliced
- 1 tablespoon dill, chopped

Directions:
1. In a bowl, mix the cucumber with the onions, vinegar and the dill, toss well and keep in the fridge for 1 hour before serving as a side salad.

Nutrition: calories 182, fat 3.5, fiber 4.5, carbs 8.5, protein 4.5

Herbed Cucumber and Avocado Mix

Preparation time: 10 minutes
Cooking time: 0 minutes
Servings: 4
Ingredients:
- 2 cucumbers, sliced
- 2 avocados, pitted, peeled and cubed
- 1 tablespoon lemon juice
- 3 tablespoons olive oil
- 2 teaspoons balsamic vinegar
- 1 teaspoon dill, dried
- 1 tablespoon cilantro, chopped
- 1 tablespoon chives, chopped
- 1 tablespoon basil, chopped
- 1 tablespoon oregano, chopped

Directions:
1. In a bowl, mix the cucumbers with the avocados with the rest of the ingredients, toss and serve as a side dish.

Nutrition: calories 343, fat 9.6, fiber 2.5, carbs 16.5, protein 7.4

Basil Bell Peppers and Cucumber Mix

Preparation time: 5 minutes
Cooking time: 0 minutes
Servings: 6
Ingredients:
- 1 red bell pepper, cut into strips
- 1 green bell pepper, cut into strips
- 2 cucumbers, sliced
- ½ cup balsamic vinegar
- 2 tablespoons olive oil
- 1 tablespoon sesame seeds, toasted
- 1 tablespoon basil, chopped

Directions:
1. In a bowl, combine the bell peppers with the cucumber and the rest of the ingredients except the sesame seeds and toss.
2. Sprinkle the sesame seeds, divide the mix between plates and serve as a side dish.

Nutrition: calories 226, fat 8.7, fiber 3.4, carbs 14.4, protein 5.6

Fennel and Walnuts Salad

Preparation time: 5 minutes
Cooking time: 0 minutes
Servings: 4
Ingredients:
- 8 dates, pitted and sliced
- 2 fennel bulbs, sliced
- 2 tablespoons chives, chopped
- ½ cup walnuts, chopped
- 2 tablespoons lime juice
- 2 tablespoons olive oil
- Salt and black pepper to the taste

Directions:
1. In a salad bowl, combine the fennel with dates and the rest of the ingredients, toss, divide between plates and serve as a side salad.

Nutrition: calories 200, fat 7.6, fiber 2.4, carbs 14.5, protein 4.3

Tomatoes and Black Beans Mix

Preparation time: 10 minutes
Cooking time: 0 minutes
Servings: 4
Ingredients:
- 15 ounces canned black beans, drained and rinsed
- 1 cup cherry tomatoes, halved
- 2 spring onions, chopped
- 3 tablespoons olive oil
- 1 and ½ teaspoons orange zest, grated
- 1 teaspoon honey
- Salt and black pepper to the taste
- ½ teaspoon cumin, ground
- 1 tablespoon lime juice

Directions:
1. In a bowl, combine the beans with cherry tomatoes, onions and the rest of the ingredients, toss and keep in the fridge for 10 minutes before serving as a side dish.

Nutrition: calories 284, fat 7.5, fiber 15.3, carbs 25.5, protein 12.4

Herbed Beets and Scallions Salad

Preparation time: 10 minutes
Cooking time: 0 minutes
Servings: 8
Ingredients:
- 4 red beets, cooked, peeled and sliced
- 6 scallions, chopped
- Zest of 1 lemon, grated
- 2 cups mixed basil with mint, parsley and cilantro, chopped
- ¼ cup balsamic vinegar
- 2 teaspoons poppy seeds
- 1 and ½ tablespoons olive oil
- Salt and black pepper to the taste

Directions:

1. In a salad bowl, combine the beets with the scallions, lemon zest and the rest of the ingredients, toss, keep in the fridge for 10 minutes and serve as a side salad.

Nutrition: calories 283, fat 11.4, fiber 3.5, carbs 13.5, protein 6.5

Tomatoes and Endives Mix

Preparation time: 10 minutes
Cooking time: 20 minutes
Servings: 4
Ingredients:
- 4 endives, shredded
- 14 ounces canned tomatoes, chopped
- Salt and black pepper to the taste
- 2 garlic cloves, minced
- ½ teaspoon red pepper, crushed
- 3 tablespoons olive oil
- 1 tablespoon oregano, chopped
- 2 tablespoons parmesan, grated
- 1 tablespoon cilantro, chopped

Directions:
1. Heat up a pan with the oil over medium heat, add the garlic and the red pepper and cook for 2-3 minutes.
2. Add the endives, tomatoes, salt, pepper and the oregano, stir and sauté for 15 minutes more.
3. Add the remaining ingredients, toss, cook for 2 minutes, divide the mix between plates and serve as a side dish.

Nutrition: calories 232, fat 7.5, fiber 3.5, carbs 14.3, protein 4.5

Yogurt Peppers Mix

Preparation time: 10 minutes
Cooking time: 15 minutes
Servings: 4
Ingredients:
- 2 red bell peppers, cut into thick strips
- 2 tablespoons olive oil
- 3 shallots, chopped
- 3 garlic cloves, minced
- Salt and black pepper to the taste
- ½ cup Greek yogurt
- 1 tablespoon cilantro, chopped

Directions:
1. Heat up a pan with the oil over medium heat, add the shallots and garlic, stir and cook for 5 minutes.
2. Add the rest of the ingredients, toss, cook for 10 minutes more, divide the mix between plates and serve as a side dish.

Nutrition: calories 274, fat 11, fiber 3.5, protein 13.3, carbs 6.5

Basil Artichokes

Preparation time: 10 minutes
Cooking time: 12 minutes
Servings: 4
Ingredients:

- 1 red onion, chopped
- 2 garlic cloves, minced
- Salt and black pepper to the taste
- ½ cup veggie stock
- 10 ounces canned artichoke hearts, drained
- 1 tablespoon olive oil
- 1 teaspoon lemon juice
- 2 tablespoons basil, chopped

Directions:
1. Heat up a pan with the oil over medium high heat, add the onion and the garlic, stir and sauté for 2 minutes.
2. Add the artichokes and the rest of the ingredients, toss, cook for 10 minutes more, divide between plates and serve as a side dish.

Nutrition: calories 105, fat 7.6, fiber 3, carbs 6.7, protein 2.5

Broccoli and Roasted Peppers

Preparation time: 10 minutes
Cooking time: 10 minutes
Servings: 4
Ingredients:
- 1 pound broccoli florets
- 2 garlic cloves, minced
- 1 tablespoon olive oil
- ¼ cup roasted peppers, chopped
- 2 tablespoons balsamic vinegar
- Salt and black pepper to the taste
- 1 tablespoon cilantro, chopped

Directions:
1. Heat up a pan with the oil over medium high heat, add the garlic and the peppers and cook for 2 minutes.
2. Add the broccoli and the rest of the ingredients, toss, cook over medium heat for 8 minutes more, divide between plates and serve as a side dish.

Nutrition: calories 193, fat 5.6, fiber 3.45, carbs 8.6, protein 4.5

Cauliflower Quinoa

Preparation time: 5 minutes
Cooking time: 10 minutes
Servings: 4
Ingredients:
- 1 and ½ cups quinoa, coked
- 3 tablespoons olive oil
- 3 cups cauliflower florets
- 2 spring onions, chopped
- Salt and pepper to the taste
- 1 tablespoon red wine vinegar
- 1 tablespoon parsley, chopped
- 1 tablespoon chives, chopped

Directions:
1. Heat up a pan with the oil over medium-high heat, add the spring onions and cook for 2 minutes.
2. Add the cauliflower, quinoa and the rest of the ingredients, toss, cook over medium heat for 8-9 minutes, divide between plates and serve as a side dish.

Nutrition: calories 220, fat 16.7, fiber 5.6, carbs 6.8, protein 5.4

Mixed Veggies and Chard

Preparation time: 10 minutes
Cooking time: 20 minutes
Servings: 4
Ingredients:
- ½ cup celery, chopped
- ½ cup carrot, chopped
- ½ cup red onion, chopped
- ½ cup red bell pepper, chopped
- 1 tablespoon olive oil
- 1 cup veggie stock
- ½ cup black olives, pitted and chopped
- 10 ounces ruby chard, torn
- Salt and black pepper to the taste
- 1 teaspoon balsamic vinegar

Directions:
1. Heat up a pan with the oil over medium-high heat, add the celery, carrot, onion, bell pepper, salt and pepper, stir and sauté for 5 minutes.
2. Add the rest of the ingredients, toss, cook over medium heat for 15 minutes more, divide between plates and serve as a side dish.

Nutrition: calories 150, fat 6.7, fiber 2.6, carbs 6.8, protein 5.4

Spicy Broccoli and Almonds

Preparation time: 10 minutes
Cooking time: 30 minutes
Servings: 4
Ingredients:
- 1 broccoli head, florets separated
- 2 garlic cloves, minced
- 1 tablespoon olive oil
- 1 tablespoon chili powder
- Salt and black pepper to the taste
- 1 tablespoon mint, chopped
- 2 tablespoons almonds, toasted and chopped

Directions:
1. In a roasting pan, combine the broccoli with the garlic, oil and the rest of the ingredients, toss, introduce in the oven and cook at 390 degrees F for 30 minutes.
2. Divide the mix between plates and serve as a side dish.

Nutrition: calories 156, fat 5.4, fiber 1.2, carbs 4.3, protein 2

Lemony Carrots

Preparation time: 10 minutes
Cooking time: 40 minutes
Servings: 4
Ingredients:
- 3 tablespoons olive oil
- 2 pounds baby carrots, trimmed
- Salt and black pepper to the taste
- ½ teaspoon lemon zest, grated
- 1 tablespoon lemon juice

- 1/3 cup Greek yogurt
- 1 garlic clove, minced
- 1 teaspoon cumin, ground
- 1 tablespoon dill, chopped

Directions:
1. In a roasting pan, combine the carrots with the oil, salt, pepper and the rest of the ingredients except the dill, toss and bake at 400 degrees F for 20 minutes.
2. Reduce the temperature to 375 degrees F and cook for 20 minutes more.
3. Divide the mix between plates, sprinkle the dill on top and serve.

Nutrition: calories 192, fat 5.4, fiber 3.4, carbs 7.3, protein 5.6

Oregano Potatoes

Preparation time: 10 minutes
Cooking time: 40 minutes
Servings: 4
Ingredients:
- 6 red potatoes, peeled and cut into wedges
- Salt and black pepper to the taste
- 2 tablespoons olive oil
- 1 teaspoon lemon zest, grated
- 1 teaspoon oregano, dried
- 1 tablespoon chives, chopped
- ½ cup chicken stock

Directions:
1. In a roasting pan, combine the potatoes with salt, pepper, the oil and the rest of the ingredients except the chives, toss, introduce in the oven and cook at 425 degrees F for 40 minutes.
2. Divide the mix between plates, sprinkle the chives on top and serve as a side dish.

Nutrition: calories 245, fat 4.5, fiber 2.8, carbs 7.1, protein 6.4

Baby Squash and Lentils Mix

Preparation time: 10 minutes
Cooking time: 10 minutes
Servings: 4
Ingredients:
- 2 tablespoons olive oil
- ½ teaspoon sweet paprika
- 10 ounces baby squash, sliced
- 1 tablespoon balsamic vinegar
- 15 ounces canned lentils, drained and rinsed
- Salt and black pepper to the taste
- 1 tablespoon dill, chopped

Directions:
1. Heat up a pan with the oil over medium heat, add the squash, lentils and the rest of the ingredients, toss and cook over medium heat for 10 minutes.
2. Divide the mix between plates and serve as a side dish.

Nutrition: calories 438, fat 8.4, fiber 32.4, carbs 65.5, protein 22.4

Parmesan Quinoa and Mushrooms

Preparation time: 10 minutes
Cooking time: 20 minutes
Servings: 4
Ingredients:
1 cup quinoa, cooked
½ cup chicken stock
2 tablespoons olive oil
6 ounces white mushrooms, sliced
1 teaspoon garlic, minced
Salt and black pepper to the taste
½ cup parmesan, grated
2 tablespoons cilantro, chopped

Directions:
1. Heat up a pan with the oil over medium heat, add the garlic and mushrooms, stir and sauté for 10 minutes.
2. Add the quinoa and the rest of the ingredients, toss, cook over medium heat for 10 minutes more, divide between plates and serve as a side dish.

Nutrition: calories 233, fat 9.5, fiber 6.4, carbs 27.4, protein 12.5

Chives Rice Mix

Preparation time: 5 minutes
Cooking time: 5 minutes
Servings: 4
Ingredients:
- 3 tablespoons avocado oil
- 1 cup Arborio rice, cooked
- 2 tablespoons chives, chopped
- Salt and black pepper to the taste
- 2 teaspoons lemon juice

Directions:
1. Heat up a pan with the avocado oil over medium high heat, add the rice and the rest of the ingredients, toss, cook for 5 minutes, divide the mix between plates and serve as a side dish.

Nutrition: calories 236, fat 9, fiber 12.4, carbs 17.5, protein 4.5

Green Beans and Peppers Mix

Preparation time: 10 minutes
Cooking time: 10 minutes
Servings: 4
Ingredients:
- 2 tablespoons olive oil
- 1 and ½ pounds green beans, trimmed and halved
- Salt and black pepper to the taste
- 2 red bell peppers, cut into strips
- 1 tablespoon lime juice
- 2 tablespoons rosemary, chopped
- 1 tablespoon dill, chopped

Directions:
1. Heat up a pan with the oil over medium heat, add the bell peppers and the green beans, toss and cook for 5 minutes.

2. Add the rest of the ingredients, toss, cook for 5 minutes more, divide between plates and serve as a side dish.
Nutrition: calories 222, fat 8.6, fiber 3.4, carbs 8.6, protein 3.4

Garlic Snap Peas Mix

Preparation time: 10 minutes
Cooking time: 10 minutes
Servings: 4
Ingredients:
- ½ cup walnuts, chopped
- 2 teaspoons lime juice
- ¼ cup olive oil
- 1 and ½ teaspoons garlic, minced
- ½ cup veggie stock
- 1 pound sugar snap peas
- Salt and black pepper to the taste
- 1 tablespoon chives, chopped

Directions:
1. Heat up a pan with the stock over medium heat, add the snap peas and cook for 5 minutes.
2. Add the rest of the ingredients except the chives, cook for 5 minutes more and divide between plates.
3. Sprinkle the chives on top and serve as a side dish.
Nutrition: calories 200, fat 7.6, fiber 3.5, carbs 8.5, protein 4.3

Corn and Olives

Preparation time: 5 minutes
Cooking time: 0 minutes
Servings: 4
Ingredients:
- 2 cups corn
- 4 ounces green olives, pitted and halved
- ½ teaspoon balsamic vinegar
- 1 tablespoon oregano, chopped
- 1 teaspoon thyme, chopped
- Salt and black pepper to the taste
- 2 tablespoons extra virgin olive oil

Directions:
1. In a bowl, combine the corn with the olives and the rest of the ingredients, toss and serve as a side dish.
Nutrition: calories 154, fat 10, fiber 3.4, carbs 17, protein 9.3

Rosemary Red Quinoa

Preparation time: 10 minutes
Cooking time: 25 minutes
Servings: 6
Ingredients:
- 4 cups chicken stock
- 2 cups red quinoa, rinsed
- 1 red onion, chopped
- 2 tablespoons olive oil
- 1 tablespoon garlic, minced
- 1 teaspoon lemon zest, grated

- 2 tablespoons lemon juice
- Salt and black pepper to the taste
- 2 tablespoons rosemary, chopped

Directions:
1. Heat up a pan with the oil over medium heat, add the onion and the garlic and sauté for 5 minutes.
2. Add the quinoa, the stock and the rest of the ingredients, bring to a simmer and cook for 20 minutes stirring from time to time.
3. Divide the mix between plates and serve.
Nutrition: calories 193, fat 7.9, fiber 1.4, carbs 5.4, protein 1.3

Thyme Corn and Cheese Mix

Preparation time: 5 minutes
Cooking time: 0 minutes
Servings: 4
Ingredients:
- 1 tablespoon olive oil
- 1 teaspoon thyme, chopped
- 1 cup scallions, sliced
- 2 cups corn
- Salt and black pepper to the taste
- 2 tablespoons blue cheese, crumbled
- 1 tablespoon chives, chopped

Directions:
1. In a salad bowl, combine the corn with scallions, thyme and the rest of the ingredients, toss, divide between plates and serve.
Nutrition: calories 183, fat 5.5, fiber 7.5, carbs 14.5

Olives and Carrots Sauté

Preparation time: 10 minutes
Cooking time: 20 minutes
Servings: 4
Ingredients:
- 1 tablespoon green olives, pitted and sliced
- 3 tablespoons olive oil
- 2 teaspoons capers, drained and chopped
- ½ teaspoon lemon zest, grated
- 1 and ½ teaspoons balsamic vinegar
- ¼ teaspoon rosemary, dried
- ¼ cup veggie stock
- Salt and black pepper to the taste
- 2 pounds carrots, sliced
- 2 spring onions, chopped
- 1 tablespoon parsley, chopped

Directions:
1. Heat up a pan with the oil over medium heat, add the carrots and brown for 5 minutes.
2. Add green olives, capers and the rest of the ingredients except the parsley and the chives, stir and cook over medium heat for 15 minutes.
3. Add the chives and parsley, toss, divide the mix between plates and serve as a side dish.
Nutrition: calories 244, fat 11, fiber 3.5, carbs 5.6, protein 6.3

Lemon Endives

Preparation time: 10 minutes

Cooking time: 35 minutes
Servings: 4
Ingredients:
- Juice of 1 and ½ lemons
- Salt and black pepper to the taste
- 3 tablespoons olive oil
- ¼ cup veggie stock
- 4 endives, halved lengthwise
- 1 tablespoon dill, chopped

Directions:
1. In a roasting pan, combine the endives with the rest of the ingredients, introduce in the oven and cook at 375 degrees F for 35 minutes.
2. Divide the endives between plates and serve as a side dish.

Nutrition: calories 221, fat 5.4, fiber 6.4, carbs 15.4, protein 14.3

Leeks Sauté

Preparation time: 10 minutes
Cooking time: 15 minutes
Servings: 4
Ingredients:
- 2 pounds leeks, sliced
- 2 tablespoons chicken stock
- 2 tablespoons tomato paste
- 1 tablespoon olive oil
- 2 tablespoons thyme, chopped
- Salt and black pepper to the taste

Directions:
1. Heat up a pan with the oil over medium heat, add the leeks and brown for 5 minutes.
2. Add the rest of the ingredients, toss, increase the heat to medium-high and cook for 10 minutes more.
3. Divide everything between plates and serve as a side dish.

Nutrition: calories 200, fat 11.4, fiber 5.6, carbs 16.4, protein 3.6

Snack and Appetizer Recipes

Meatballs Platter

Preparation time: 10 minutes
Cooking time: 15 minutes
Servings: 4
Ingredients:
- 1 pound beef meat, ground
- ¼ cup panko breadcrumbs
- A pinch of salt and black pepper
- 3 tablespoons red onion, grated
- ¼ cup parsley, chopped
- 2 garlic cloves, minced
- 2 tablespoons lemon juice
- Zest of 1 lemon, grated
- 1 egg
- ½ teaspoon cumin, ground
- ½ teaspoon coriander, ground
- ¼ teaspoon cinnamon powder
- 2 ounces feta cheese, crumbled
- Cooking spray

Directions:
1. In a bowl, mix the beef with the breadcrumbs, salt, pepper and the rest of the ingredients except the cooking spray, stir well and shape medium balls out of this mix.
2. Arrange the meatballs on a baking sheet lined with parchment paper, grease them with cooking spray and bake at 450 degrees F for 15 minutes.
3. Arrange the meatballs on a platter and serve as an appetizer.
Nutrition: calories 300, fat 15.4, fiber 6.4, carbs 22.4, protein 35

Yogurt Dip

Preparation time: 10 minutes
Cooking time: 0 minutes
Servings: 6
Ingredients:
- 2 cups Greek yogurt
- 2 tablespoons pistachios, toasted and chopped
- A pinch of salt and white pepper
- 2 tablespoons mint, chopped
- 1 tablespoon kalamata olives, pitted and chopped
- ¼ cup za'atar spice
- ¼ cup pomegranate seeds
- 1/3 cup olive oil

Directions:
1. In a bowl, combine the yogurt with the pistachios and the rest of the ingredients, whisk well, divide into small cups and serve with pita chips on the side.
Nutrition: calories 294, fat 18, fiber 1, carbs 21, protein 10

Tomato Bruschetta

Preparation time: 10 minutes
Cooking time: 10 minutes
Servings: 6

Ingredients:
- 1 baguette, sliced
- 1/3 cup basil, chopped
- 6 tomatoes, cubed
- 2 garlic cloves, minced
- A pinch of salt and black pepper
- 1 teaspoon olive oil
- 1 tablespoon balsamic vinegar
- ½ teaspoon garlic powder
- Cooking spray

Directions:
1. Arrange the baguette slices on a baking sheet lined with parchment paper, grease them with cooking spray and bake at 400 degrees F for 10 minutes.
2. In a bowl, mix the tomatoes with the basil and the remaining ingredients, toss well and leave aside for 10 minutes.
3. Divide the tomato mix on each baguette slice, arrange them all on a platter and serve.
Nutrition: calories 162, fat 4 fiber 7, carbs 29, protein 4

Artichoke Flatbread

Preparation time: 10 minutes
Cooking time: 15 minutes
Servings: 4
Ingredients:
- 5 tablespoons olive oil
- 2 garlic cloves, minced
- 2 tablespoons parsley, chopped
- 2 round whole wheat flatbreads
- 4 tablespoons parmesan, grated
- ½ cup mozzarella cheese, grated
- 14 ounces canned artichokes, drained and quartered
- 1 cup baby spinach, chopped
- ½ cup cherry tomatoes, halved
- ½ teaspoon basil, dried
- Salt and black pepper to the taste

Directions:
1. In a bowl, mix the parsley with the garlic and 4 tablespoons oil, whisk well and spread this over the flatbreads.
2. Sprinkle the mozzarella and half of the parmesan.
3. In a bowl, mix the artichokes with the spinach, tomatoes, basil, salt, pepper and the rest of the oil, toss and divide over the flatbreads as well.
4. Sprinkle the rest of the parmesan on top, arrange the flatbreads on a baking sheet lined with parchment paper and bake at 425 degrees F for 15 minutes.
5. Serve as an appetizer.
Nutrition: calories 223, fat 11.2, fiber 5.34, carbs 15.5, protein 7.4

Red Pepper Tapenade

Preparation time: 10 minutes
Cooking time: 0 minutes

Servings: 4
Ingredients:
- 7 ounces roasted red peppers, chopped
- ½ cup parmesan, grated
- 1/3 cup parsley, chopped
- 14 ounces canned artichokes, drained and chopped
- 3 tablespoons olive oil
- ¼ cup capers, drained
- 1 and ½ tablespoons lemon juice
- 2 garlic cloves, minced

Directions:
1.   In your blender, combine the red peppers with the parmesan and the rest of the ingredients and pulse well.
2.   Divide into cups and serve as a snack.

Nutrition: calories 200, fat 5.6, fiber 4.5, carbs 12.4, protein 4.6

Coriander Falafel

Preparation time: 10 minutes
Cooking time: 10 minutes
Servings: 8
Ingredients:
- 1 cup canned garbanzo beans, drained and rinsed
- 1 bunch parsley leaves
- 1 yellow onion, chopped
- 5 garlic cloves, minced
- 1 teaspoon coriander, ground
- A pinch of salt and black pepper
- ¼ teaspoon cayenne pepper
- ¼ teaspoon baking soda
- ¼ teaspoon cumin powder
- 1 teaspoon lemon juice
- 3 tablespoons tapioca flour
- Olive oil for frying

Directions:
1.   In your food processor, combine the beans with the parsley, onion and the rest the ingredients except the oil and the flour and pulse well.
2.   Transfer the mix to a bowl, add the flour, stir well, shape 16 balls out of this mix and flatten them a bit.
3.   Heat up a pan with some oil over medium-high heat, add the falafels, cook them for 5 minutes on each side, transfer to paper towels, drain excess grease, arrange them on a platter and serve as an appetizer.

Nutrition: calories 112, fat 6.2, fiber 2, carbs 12.3, protein 3.1

Red Pepper Hummus

Preparation time: 10 minutes
Cooking time: 0 minutes
Servings: 6
Ingredients:
- 6 ounces roasted red peppers, peeled and chopped

- 16 ounces canned chickpeas, drained and rinsed
- ¼ cup Greek yogurt
- 3 tablespoons tahini paste
- Juice of 1 lemon
- 3 garlic cloves, minced
- 1 tablespoon olive oil
- A pinch of salt and black pepper
- 1 tablespoon parsley, chopped

Directions:
1.   In your food processor, combine the red peppers with the rest of the ingredients except the oil and the parsley and pulse well.
2.   Add the oil, pulse again, divide into cups, sprinkle the parsley on top and serve as a party spread.

Nutrition: calories 255, fat 11.4, fiber 4.5, carbs 17.4, protein 6.5

White Bean Dip

Preparation time: 10 minutes
Cooking time: 0 minutes
Servings: 4
Ingredients:
- 15 ounces canned white beans, drained and rinsed
- 6 ounces canned artichoke hearts, drained and quartered
- 4 garlic cloves, minced
- 1 tablespoon basil, chopped
- 2 tablespoons olive oil
- Juice of ½ lemon
- Zest of ½ lemon, grated
- Salt and black pepper to the taste

Directions:
1.   In your food processor, combine the beans with the artichokes and the rest of the ingredients except the oil and pulse well.
2.   Add the oil gradually, pulse the mix again, divide into cups and serve as a party dip.

Nutrition: calories 274, fat 11.7, fiber 6.5, carbs 18.5, protein 16.5

Hummus with Ground Lamb

Preparation time: 10 minutes
Cooking time: 15 minutes
Servings: 8
Ingredients:
- 10 ounces hummus
- 12 ounces lamb meat, ground
- ½ cup pomegranate seeds
- ¼ cup parsley, chopped
- 1 tablespoon olive oil
- Pita chips for serving

Directions:
1.   Heat up a pan with the oil over medium-high heat, add the meat, and brown for 15 minutes stirring often.
2.   Spread the hummus on a platter, spread the ground lamb all over, also spread the pomegranate

seeds and the parsley and sere with pita chips as a snack.
Nutrition: calories 133, fat 9.7, fiber 1.7, carbs 6.4, protein 5.4

Eggplant Dip

Preparation time: 10 minutes
Cooking time: 40 minutes
Servings: 4
Ingredients:
- 1 eggplant, poked with a fork
- 2 tablespoons tahini paste
- 2 tablespoons lemon juice
- 2 garlic cloves, minced
- 1 tablespoon olive oil
- Salt and black pepper to the taste
- 1 tablespoon parsley, chopped

Directions:
1. Put the eggplant in a roasting pan, bake at 400 degrees F for 40 minutes, cool down, peel and transfer to your food processor.
2. Add the rest of the ingredients except the parsley, pulse well, divide into small bowls and serve as an appetizer with the parsley sprinkled on top.
Nutrition: calories 121, fat 4.3, fiber 1, carbs 1.4, protein 4.3

Veggie Fritters

Preparation time: 10 minutes
Cooking time: 10 minutes
Servings: 8
Ingredients:
- 2 garlic cloves, minced
- 2 yellow onions, chopped
- 4 scallions, chopped
- 2 carrots, grated
- 2 teaspoons cumin, ground
- ½ teaspoon turmeric powder
- Salt and black pepper to the taste
- ¼ teaspoon coriander, ground
- 2 tablespoons parsley, chopped
- ¼ teaspoon lemon juice
- ½ cup almond flour
- 2 beets, peeled and grated
- 2 eggs, whisked
- ¼ cup tapioca flour
- 3 tablespoons olive oil

Directions:
1. In a bowl, combine the garlic with the onions, scallions and the rest of the ingredients except the oil, stir well and shape medium fritters out of this mix.
2. Heat up a pan with the oil over medium-high heat, add the fritters, cook for 5 minutes on each side, arrange on a platter and serve.
Nutrition: calories 209, fat 11.2, fiber 3, carbs 4.4, protein 4.8

Bulgur Lamb Meatballs

Preparation time: 10 minutes
Cooking time: 15 minutes

Servings: 6
Ingredients:
- 1 and ½ cups Greek yogurt
- ½ teaspoon cumin, ground
- 1 cup cucumber, shredded
- ½ teaspoon garlic, minced
- A pinch of salt and black pepper
- 1 cup bulgur
- 2 cups water
- 1 pound lamb, ground
- ¼ cup parsley, chopped
- ¼ cup shallots, chopped
- ½ teaspoon allspice, ground
- ½ teaspoon cinnamon powder
- 1 tablespoon olive oil

Directions:
1. In a bowl, combine the bulgur with the water, cover the bowl, leave aside for 10 minutes, drain and transfer to a bowl.
2. Add the meat, the yogurt and the rest of the ingredients except the oil, stir well and shape medium meatballs out of this mix.
3. Heat up a pan with the oil over medium-high heat, add the meatballs, cook them for 7 minutes on each side, arrange them all on a platter and serve as an appetizer.
Nutrition: calories 300, fat 9.6, fiber 4.6, carbs 22.6, protein 6.6

Cucumber Bites

Preparation time: 10 minutes
Cooking time: 0 minutes
Servings: 12
Ingredients:
- 1 English cucumber, sliced into 32 rounds
- 10 ounces hummus
- 16 cherry tomatoes, halved
- 1 tablespoon parsley, chopped
- 1 ounce feta cheese, crumbled

Directions:
1. Spread the hummus on each cucumber round, divide the tomato halves on each, sprinkle the cheese and parsley on to and serve as an appetizer.
Nutrition: calories 162, fat 3.4, fiber 2, carbs 6.4, protein 2.4

Stuffed Avocado

Preparation time: 10 minutes
Cooking time: 0 minutes
Servings: 2
Ingredients:
- 1 avocado, halved and pitted
- 10 ounces canned tuna, drained
- 2 tablespoons sun-dried tomatoes, chopped
- 1 and ½ tablespoon basil pesto
- 2 tablespoons black olives, pitted and chopped
- Salt and black pepper to the taste
- 2 teaspoons pine nuts, toasted and chopped
- 1 tablespoon basil, chopped

Directions:

1.   In a bowl, combine the tuna with the sun-dried tomatoes and the rest of the ingredients except the avocado and stir.
2.   Stuff the avocado halves with the tuna mix and serve as an appetizer.
Nutrition: calories 233, fat 9, fiber 3.5, carbs 11.4, protein 5.6

Wrapped Plums

Preparation time: 5 minutes
Cooking time: 0 minutes
Servings: 8
Ingredients:
- 2 ounces prosciutto, cut into 16 pieces
- 4 plums, quartered
- 1 tablespoon chives, chopped
- A pinch of red pepper flakes, crushed

Directions:
1.   Wrap each plum quarter in a prosciutto slice, arrange them all on a platter, sprinkle the chives and pepper flakes all over and serve.
Nutrition: calories 30, fat 1, fiber 0, carbs 4, protein 2

Cucumber Sandwich Bites

Preparation time: 5 minutes
Cooking time: 0 minutes
Servings: 12
Ingredients:
- 1 cucumber, sliced
- 8 slices whole wheat bread
- 2 tablespoons cream cheese, soft
- 1 tablespoon chives, chopped
- ¼ cup avocado, peeled, pitted and mashed
- 1 teaspoon mustard
- Salt and black pepper to the taste

Directions:
1.   Spread the mashed avocado on each bread slice, also spread the rest of the ingredients except the cucumber slices.
2.   Divide the cucumber slices on the bread slices, cut each slice in thirds, arrange on a platter and serve as an appetizer.
Nutrition: calories 187, fat 12.4, fiber 2.1, carbs 4.5, protein 8.2

Cucumber Rolls

Preparation time: 5 minutes
Cooking time: 0 minutes
Servings: 6
Ingredients:
- 1 big cucumber, sliced lengthwise
- 1 tablespoon parsley, chopped
- 8 ounces canned tuna, drained and mashed
- Salt and black pepper to the taste
- 1 teaspoon lime juice

Directions:
1.   Arrange cucumber slices on a working surface, divide the rest of the ingredients, and roll.
2.   Arrange all the rolls on a platter and serve as an appetizer.

Nutrition: calories 200, fat 6, fiber 3.4, carbs 7.6, protein 3.5

Olives and Cheese Stuffed Tomatoes

Preparation time: 10 minutes
Cooking time: 0 minutes
Servings: 24
Ingredients:
- 24 cherry tomatoes, top cut off and insides scooped out
- 2 tablespoons olive oil
- ¼ teaspoon red pepper flakes
- ½ cup feta cheese, crumbled
- 2 tablespoons black olive paste
- ¼ cup mint, torn

Directions:
1.   In a bowl, mix the olives paste with the rest of the ingredients except the cherry tomatoes and whisk well.
2.   Stuff the cherry tomatoes with this mix, arrange them all on a platter and serve as an appetizer.
Nutrition: calories 136, fat 8.6, fiber 4.8, carbs 5.6, protein 5.1

Tomato Salsa

Preparation time: 5 minutes
Cooking time: 0 minutes
Servings: 6
Ingredients:
- 1 garlic clove, minced
- 4 tablespoons olive oil
- 5 tomatoes, cubed
- 1 tablespoon balsamic vinegar
- ¼ cup basil, chopped
- 1 tablespoon parsley, chopped
- 1 tablespoon chives, chopped
- Salt and black pepper to the taste
- Pita chips for serving

Directions:
1.   In a bowl, mix the tomatoes with the garlic and the rest of the ingredients except the pita chips, stir, divide into small cups and serve with the pita chips on the side.
Nutrition: calories 160, fat 13.7, fiber 5.5, carbs 10.1, protein 2.2

Chili Mango and Watermelon Salsa

Preparation time: 5 minutes
Cooking time: 0 minutes
Servings: 12
Ingredients:
- 1 red tomato, chopped
- Salt and black pepper to the taste
- 1 cup watermelon, seedless, peeled and cubed
- 1 red onion, chopped
- 2 mangos, peeled and chopped
- 2 chili peppers, chopped
- ¼ cup cilantro, chopped
- 3 tablespoons lime juice
- Pita chips for serving

Directions:
1. In a bowl, mix the tomato with the watermelon, the onion and the rest of the ingredients except the pita chips and toss well.
2. Divide the mix into small cups and serve with pita chips on the side.
Nutrition: calories 62, fat 4.7, fiber 1.3, carbs 3.9, protein 2.3

Creamy Spinach and Shallots Dip

Preparation time: 10 minutes
Cooking time: 0 minutes
Servings: 4
Ingredients:
- 1 pound spinach, roughly chopped
- 2 shallots, chopped
- 2 tablespoons mint, chopped
- ¾ cup cream cheese, soft
- Salt and black pepper to the taste

Directions:
1. In a blender, combine the spinach with the shallots and the rest of the ingredients, and pulse well.
2. Divide into small bowls and serve as a party dip.
Nutrition: calories 204, fat 11.5, fiber 3.1, carbs 4.2, protein 5.9

Feta Artichoke Dip

Preparation time: 10 minutes
Cooking time: 30 minutes
Servings: 8
Ingredients:
- 8 ounces artichoke hearts, drained and quartered
- ¾ cup basil, chopped
- ¾ cup green olives, pitted and chopped
- 1 cup parmesan cheese, grated
- 5 ounces feta cheese, crumbled

Directions:
1. In your food processor, mix the artichokes with the basil and the rest of the ingredients, pulse well, and transfer to a baking dish.
2. Introduce in the oven, bake at 375 degrees F for 30 minutes and serve as a party dip.
Nutrition: calories 186, fat 12.4, fiber 0.9, carbs 2.6, protein 1.5

Avocado Dip

Preparation time: 5 minutes
Cooking time: 0 minutes
Servings: 8
Ingredients:
- ½ cup heavy cream
- 1 green chili pepper, chopped
- Salt and pepper to the taste
- 4 avocados, pitted, peeled and chopped
- 1 cup cilantro, chopped
- ¼ cup lime juice

Directions:

1. In a blender, combine the cream with the avocados and the rest of the ingredients and pulse well.
2. Divide the mix into bowls and serve cold as a party dip.
Nutrition: calories 200, fat 14.5, fiber 3.8, carbs 8.1, protein 7.6

Goat Cheese and Chives Spread

Preparation time: 10 minutes
Cooking time: 0 minutes
Servings: 4
Ingredients:
- 2 ounces goat cheese, crumbled
- ¾ cup sour cream
- 2 tablespoons chives, chopped
- 1 tablespoon lemon juice
- Salt and black pepper to the taste
- 2 tablespoons extra virgin olive oil

Directions:
1. In a bowl, mix the goat cheese with the cream and the rest of the ingredients and whisk really well.
2. Keep in the fridge for 10 minutes and serve as a party spread.
Nutrition: calories 220, fat 11.5, fiber 4.8, carbs 8.9, protein 5.6

Chickpeas Salsa

Preparation time: 5 minutes
Cooking time: 0 minutes
Servings: 6
Ingredients:
- 4 spring onions, chopped
- 1 cup baby spinach
- 15 ounces canned chickpeas, drained and rinsed
- Salt and black pepper to the taste
- 2 tablespoons olive oil
- 2 tablespoons lemon juice
- 1 tablespoon cilantro, chopped

Directions:
1. In a bowl, mix the chickpeas with the spinach, spring onions and the rest of the ingredients, toss, divide into small cups and serve as a snack.
Nutrition: calories 224, fat 5.1, fiber 1, carbs 9.9, protein 15.1

Ginger and Cream Cheese Dip

Preparation time: 5 minutes
Cooking time: 0 minutes
Servings: 6
Ingredients:
- ½ cup ginger, grated
- 2 bunches cilantro, chopped
- 3 tablespoons balsamic vinegar
- ½ cup olive oil
- 1 and ½ cups cream cheese, soft

Directions:
1. In your blender, mix the ginger with the rest of the ingredients and pulse well.

2. Divide into small bowls and serve as a party dip.
Nutrition: calories 213, fat 4.9, fiber 4.1, carbs 8.8, protein 17.8

Walnuts Yogurt Dip
Preparation time: 5 minutes
Cooking time: 0 minutes
Servings: 8
Ingredients:
- 3 garlic cloves, minced
- 2 cups Greek yogurt
- ¼ cup dill, chopped
- 1 tablespoon chives, chopped
- ¼ cup walnuts, chopped
- Salt and black pepper to the taste

Directions:
1. In a bowl, mix the garlic with the yogurt and the rest of the ingredients, whisk well, divide into small cups and serve as a party dip.
Nutrition: calories 200, fat 6.5, fiber 4.6, carbs 15.5, protein 8.4

Herbed Goat Cheese Dip
Preparation time: 5 minutes
Cooking time: 0 minutes
Servings: 4
Ingredients:
- ¼ cup mixed parsley, chopped
- ¼ cup chives, chopped
- 8 ounces goat cheese, soft
- Salt and black pepper to the taste
- A drizzle of olive oil

Directions:
1. In your food processor mix the goat cheese with the parsley and the rest of the ingredients and pulse well.
2. Divide into small bowls and serve as a party dip.
Nutrition: calories 245, fat 11.3, fiber 4.5, carbs 8.9, protein 11.2

Scallions Dip
Preparation time: 5 minutes
Cooking time: 0 minutes
Servings: 8
Ingredients:
- 6 scallions, chopped
- 1 garlic clove, minced
- 3 tablespoons olive oil
- Salt and black pepper to the taste
- 1 tablespoon lemon juice
- 1 and ½ cups cream cheese, soft
- 2 ounces prosciutto, cooked and crumbled

Directions:
1. In a bowl, mix the scallions with the garlic and the rest of the ingredients except the prosciutto and whisk well.
2. Divide into bowls, sprinkle the prosciutto on top and serve as a party dip.
Nutrition: calories 144, fat 7.7, fiber 1.4, carbs 6.3, protein 5.5

Tomato Cream Cheese Spread
Preparation time: 5 minutes
Cooking time: 0 minutes
Servings: 6
Ingredients:
- 12 ounces cream cheese, soft
- 1 big tomato, cubed
- ¼ cup homemade mayonnaise
- 2 garlic clove, minced
- 2 tablespoons red onion, chopped
- 2 tablespoons lime juice
- Salt and black pepper to the taste

Directions:
1. In your blender, mix the cream cheese with the tomato and the rest of the ingredients, pulse well, divide into small cups and serve cold.
Nutrition: calories 204, fat 6.7, fiber 1.4, carbs 7.3, protein 4.5

Pesto Dip
Preparation time: 5 minutes
Cooking time: 0 minutes
Servings: 6
Ingredients:
- 1 cup cream cheese, soft
- 3 tablespoons basil pesto
- Salt and black pepper to the taste
- 1 cup heavy cream
- 1 tablespoon chives, chopped

Directions:
1. In a bowl, mix the cream cheese with the pesto and the rest of the ingredients and whisk well.
2. Divide into small cups and serve as a party dip.
Nutrition: calories 230, fat 14.5, fiber 4.8, carbs 6.5, protein 5.4

Vinegar Beet Bites
Preparation time: 10 minutes
Cooking time: 30 minutes
Servings: 4
Ingredients:
- 2 beets, sliced
- A pinch of sea salt and black pepper
- 1/3 cup balsamic vinegar
- 1 cup olive oil

Directions:
1. Spread the beet slices on a baking sheet lined with parchment paper, add the rest of the ingredients, toss and bake at 350 degrees F for 30 minutes.
2. Serve the beet bites cold as a snack.
Nutrition: calories 199, fat 5.4, fiber 3.5, carbs 8.5, protein 3.5

Zucchini and Olives Salsa
Preparation time: 5 minutes
Cooking time: 0 minutes
Servings: 4
Ingredients:
- ½ cup black olives, pitted and sliced
- 3 zucchinis, cut with a spiralizer

- 1 cup cherry tomatoes, halved
- Salt and black pepper to the taste
- 1 small red onion, chopped
- ½ cup feta cheese, crumbled
- ½ cup olive oil
- ¼ cup apple cider vinegar

Directions:
1. In a bowl, mix the olives with the zucchinis and the rest of the ingredients, toss, divide into small cups and serve as an appetizer.

Nutrition: calories 140, fat 14.2, fiber 1.4, carbs 3.5, protein 1.4

Strawberry and Carrots Salad

Preparation time: 5 minutes
Cooking time: 0 minutes
Servings: 4
Ingredients:
- 6 carrots, peeled and grated
- 10 strawberries, halved
- Salt and black pepper to the taste
- 2 tablespoons balsamic vinegar
- 1 tablespoon Dijon mustard
- ¼ cup lemon juice
- 2 tablespoons olive oil

Directions:
1. In a bowl, mix the carrots with the strawberries and the rest of the ingredients, toss, divide between appetizer plates and serve.

Nutrition: calories 182, fat 4.3, fiber 2.4, carbs 7.5, protein 3

Hot Squash Wedges

Preparation time: 10 minutes
Cooking time: 25 minutes
Servings: 6
Ingredients:
- 6 tablespoons olive oil
- 2 tablespoons chili paste
- 3 butternut squash, peeled and cut into wedges
- 2 tablespoons balsamic vinegar
- 1 tablespoon chives, chopped

Directions:
1. In a bowl, mix the squash wedges with the chili paste and the rest of the ingredients, toss, spread them on a baking sheet lined with parchment paper and bake at 400 degrees F for 25 minutes, flipping them from time to time.
2. Divide the wedges into bowls and serve as a snack.

Nutrition: calories 180, fat 4.2, fiber 4.4, carbs 6.5, protein 1.4

Shrimp and Cucumber Bites

Preparation time: 5 minutes
Cooking time: 0 minutes
Servings: 8
Ingredients:
- 1 big cucumber, cubed

- 1 pound shrimp, cooked, peeled, deveined and chopped
- 2 tablespoons heavy cream
- Salt and black pepper to the taste
- 12 whole grain crackers

Directions:
1. In a bowl, mix the cucumber with the rest of the ingredients except the crackers and stir well.
2. Arrange the crackers on a platter, spread the shrimp mix on each and serve.

Nutrition: calories 155, fat 8.5, fiber 4.8, carbs 11.8, protein 17.7

Salmon Rolls

Preparation time: 5 minutes
Cooking time: 0 minutes
Servings: 12
Ingredients:
- 1 big long cucumber, thinly sliced lengthwise
- 2 teaspoons lime juice
- 4 ounces cream cheese, soft
- 1 teaspoon lemon zest, grated
- Salt and black pepper to the taste
- 2 teaspoons dill, chopped
- 4 ounces smoked salmon, cut into strips

Directions:
1. Arrange cucumber slices on a working surface and top each with a salmon strip.
2. In a bowl, mix the rest of the ingredients, stir and spread over the salmon.
3. Roll the salmon and cucumber strips, arrange them on a platter and serve as an appetizer.

Nutrition: calories 245, fat 15.5, fiber 4.8, carbs 16.8, protein 17.3

Eggplant Bombs

Preparation time: 10 minutes
Cooking time: 45 minutes
Servings: 6
Ingredients:
- 4 cups eggplants, chopped
- 3 tablespoons olive oil
- 3 garlic cloves, minced
- 2 eggs, whisked
- Salt and black pepper to the taste
- 1 cup parsley, chopped
- ½ cup parmesan cheese, finely grated
- ¾ cups bread crumbs

Directions:
1. Heat up a pan with the oil over medium high heat, add the garlic and the eggplants, and cook for 15 minutes stirring often.
2. In a bowl, combine the eggplant mix with the rest of the ingredients, stir well and shape medium balls out of this mix.
3. Arrange the balls on a baking sheet lined with parchment paper and bake at 350 degrees F for 30 minutes.
4. Serve as a snack.

Nutrition: calories 224, fat 10.6, fiber 1.8, carbs 5.4, protein 3.5

Eggplant Bites

Preparation time: 10 minutes
Cooking time: 15 minutes
Servings: 8
Ingredients:

- 2 eggplants, cut into 20 slices
- 2 tablespoons olive oil
- ½ cup roasted peppers, chopped
- ½ cup kalamata olives, pitted and chopped
- 1 tablespoon lime juice
- 1 teaspoon red pepper flakes, crushed
- Salt and black pepper to the taste
- 2 tablespoons mint, chopped

Directions:
1.   In a bowl, mix the roasted peppers with the olives, half of the oil and the rest of the ingredients except the eggplant slices and stir well.
2.   Brush eggplant slices with the rest of the olive oil on both sides, place them on the preheated grill over medium high heat, cook for 7 minutes on each side and transfer them to a platter.
3.   Top each eggplant slice with roasted peppers mix and serve.
Nutrition: calories 214, fat 10.6, fiber 5.8, carbs 15.4, protein 5.4

Sage Eggplant Chips

Preparation time: 10 minutes
Cooking time: 45 minutes
Servings: 4
Ingredients:

- 1 tablespoon olive oil
- 2 eggplants, sliced
- ½ tablespoon smoked paprika
- Salt and black pepper to the taste
- ½ teaspoon turmeric powder
- ½ teaspoon onion powder
- 2 teaspoons sage, dried

Directions:
1.   In a bowl, mix the eggplant slices with the rest of the ingredients and toss well.
2.   Spread the eggplant slices on a baking sheet lined with parchment paper, bake at 360 degrees F for 45 minutes and serve cold as a snack.
Nutrition: calories 139, fat 7.1, fiber 4.1, carbs 11.3, protein 2.5

Tomato Dip

Preparation time: 10 minutes
Cooking time: 0 minutes
Servings: 4
Ingredients:

- 1 pound tomatoes, peeled and chopped
- Salt and black pepper to the taste
- 1 and ½ teaspoons balsamic vinegar
- ½ teaspoon oregano, chopped
- 3 tablespoons olive oil

- 2 garlic cloves, minced
- 3 tablespoons parsley, chopped

Directions:
1.   In a blender, combine the tomatoes with the oregano, salt, pepper and the rest of the ingredients, pulse well, divide into small cups and serve as a party dip.
Nutrition: calories 124, fat 4, fiber 2.1, carbs 3.3, protein 3.2

Oregano Avocado Salad

Preparation time: 10 minutes
Cooking time: 0 minutes
Servings: 4
Ingredients:

- A drizzle of olive oil
- 4 small avocados, pitted and cubed
- 1 teaspoon mustard
- 1 tablespoon white vinegar
- 1 tablespoon oregano, chopped
- 1 teaspoon honey
- Salt and black pepper to the taste

Directions:
1.   In a bowl, combine the avocados with the oil and the rest of the ingredients, toss, divide between appetizer plates and serve.
Nutrition: calories 244, fat 14, fiber 12.1, carbs 23.3, protein 8.2

Lentils Spread

Preparation time: 2 hours
Cooking time: 0 minutes
Servings: 12
Ingredients:

- 1 garlic clove, minced
- 12 ounces canned lentils, drained and rinsed
- 1 teaspoon oregano, dried
- ¼ teaspoon basil, dried
- 3 tablespoons olive oil
- 1 tablespoon balsamic vinegar
- Salt and black pepper to the taste

Directions:
1.   In a blender, combine the lentils with the garlic and the rest of the ingredients, pulse well, divide into bowls and serve as an appetizer.
Nutrition: calories 287, fat 9.5, fiber 3.5, carbs 15.3, protein 9.3

Chickpeas and Eggplant Bowls

Preparation time: 10 minutes
Cooking time: 10 minutes
Servings: 4
Ingredients:

- 2 eggplants, cut in half lengthwise and cubed
- 1 red onion, chopped
- Juice of 1 lime
- 1 tablespoon olive oil
- 28 ounces canned chickpeas, drained and rinsed
- 1 bunch parsley, chopped

- A pinch of salt and black pepper
- 1 tablespoon balsamic vinegar

Directions:

1.   Spread the eggplant cubes on a baking sheet lined with parchment paper, drizzle half of the oil all over, season with salt and pepper and cook at 425 degrees F for 10 minutes.

2.   Cool the eggplant down, add the rest of the ingredients, toss, divide between appetizer plates and serve.

Nutrition: calories 263, fat 12, fiber 9.3, carbs 15.4, protein 7.5

Cheese and Egg Salad

Preparation time: 10 minutes
Cooking time: 0 minutes
Servings: 4
Ingredients:

- 2 tablespoons olive oil
- 12 eggs, hard boiled, peeled and chopped
- Juice of 1 lime
- 14 ounces feta cheese, crumbled
- Salt and black pepper to the taste
- ¼ cup mustard
- ¾ cup sun-dried tomatoes, chopped
- 1 cup walnuts, chopped

Directions:

1.   In a bowl, combine the eggs with the oil, and the rest of the ingredients and stir well.

2.   Divide into small bowls and serve cold as an appetizer.

Nutrition: calories 288, fat 8, fiber 4.5, carbs 15.4, protein 6.7

Stuffed Zucchinis

Preparation time: 10 minutes
Cooking time: 40 minutes
Servings: 6
Ingredients:

- 6 zucchinis, halved lengthwise and insides scooped out
- 2 garlic cloves, minced
- 2 tablespoons oregano, chopped
- Juice of 2 lemons
- Salt and black pepper to the taste
- 2 tablespoons olive oil
- 8 ounces feta cheese, crumbed

Directions:

1.   Arrange the zucchini halves on a baking sheet lined with parchment paper, divide the cheese and the rest of the ingredients in each zucchini half and bake at 450 degrees F for 40 minutes.

2.   Arrange the stuffed zucchinis on a platter and serve as an appetizer.

Nutrition: calories

Eggplant And Capers Dip

Preparation time: 10 minutes
Cooking time: 0 minutes
Servings: 4

Ingredients:

- 1 and ½ pounds eggplants, baked, peeled and chopped
- 1 red chili pepper, chopped
- ¾ cup olive oil
- 1 red bell pepper, roasted and chopped
- 1 and ½ teaspoons capers, drained and chopped
- 1 big garlic clove, minced
- 1 bunch parsley, chopped
- Salt and black pepper to the taste

Directions:

1.   In a blender, combine the eggplants with the oil, chili pepper and the rest of the ingredients, pulse well, divide into bowls and serve as a party dip.

Nutrition: calories

Pomegranate Dip

Preparation time: 10 minutes
Cooking time: 0 minutes
Servings: 6
Ingredients:

- 1 tablespoon olive oil
- 3 garlic cloves, peeled
- 1/8 teaspoon cumin
- 6 tablespoons cold water
- ½ cup tahini paste
- ½ cup pomegranate seeds
- ¼ cup pistachios, chopped

Directions:

1.   In a blender, combine the oil with the garlic and the rest of the ingredients, pulse well, divide into cups and serve cold as a party dip.

Nutrition: calories 200, fat 1.6, fiber 5.4, carbs 8.5, protein 6.3

Lentils and Tomato Dip

Preparation time: 1 hour
Cooking time: 0 minutes
Servings: 6
Ingredients:

- 1 cup red lentils, cooked
- Salt and black pepper to the taste
- 2 tablespoons lemon juice
- 1 garlic clove, minced
- 2 tablespoons tomato paste
- 2 tablespoon cilantro, chopped
- 2 tablespoons olive oil
- 2 teaspoons cumin, ground

Directions:

1.   In your blender, combine the lentils with the lemon juice, salt, pepper and the rest of the ingredients, and pulse well.

2.   Transfer to a bowl and keep in the fridge for 1 hour before serving.

Nutrition: calories 244, fat 8, fiber 12.4, carbs 26, protein 8.5

Lentils Stuffed Potato Skins

Preparation time: 10 minutes

Cooking time: 30 minutes
Servings: 8
Ingredients:
- 16 red baby potatoes
- ¾ cup red lentils, cooked and drained
- 2 tablespoons olive oil
- 2 garlic cloves, minced
- 1 tablespoon chives, chopped
- ½ teaspoon hot chili sauce
- Salt and black pepper to the taste

Directions:
1.   Put potatoes in a pot, add water to cover them, bring to a boil over medium low heat, cook for 15 minutes, drain, cool them down, cut in halves, remove the pulp, transfer it to a blender and pulse it a bit.
2.   Add the rest of the ingredients to the blender, pulse again well and stuff the potato skins with this mix.
3.   Arrange the stuffed potatoes on a baking sheet lined with parchment paper, introduce them in the oven at 375 degrees F and bake for 15 minutes.
4.   Arrange on a platter and serve as an appetizer.
Nutrition: calories 300, fat 9.3, fiber 14.5, carbs 22.5, protein 8.5

Fish and Seafood Recipes

Fish and Orzo

Preparation time: 10 minutes
Cooking time: 35 minutes
Servings: 4
Ingredients:
- 1 teaspoon garlic, minced
- 1 teaspoon red pepper, crushed
- 2 shallots, chopped
- 1 tablespoon olive oil
- 1 teaspoon anchovy paste
- 1 tablespoon oregano, chopped
- 2 tablespoons black olives, pitted and chopped
- 2 tablespoons capers, drained
- 15 ounces canned tomatoes, crushed
- A pinch of salt and black pepper
- 4 cod fillets, boneless
- 1 ounce feta cheese, crumbled
- 1 tablespoons parsley, chopped
- 3 cups chicken stock
- 1 cup orzo pasta
- Zest of 1 lemon, grated

Directions:
1. Heat up a pan with the oil over medium heat, add the garlic, red pepper and the shallots and sauté for 5 minutes.
2. Add the anchovy paste, oregano, black olives, capers, tomatoes, salt and pepper, stir and cook for 5 minutes more.
3. Add the cod fillets, sprinkle the cheese and the parsley on top, introduce in the oven and bake at 375 degrees F for 15 minutes more.
4. Meanwhile, put the stock in a pot, bring to a boil over medium heat, add the orzo and the lemon zest, bring to a simmer, cook for 10 minutes, fluff with a fork, and divide between plates.
5. Top each serving with the fish mix and serve.
Nutrition: calories 402, fat 21, fiber 8, carbs 21, protein 31

Baked Sea Bass

Preparation time: 10 minutes
Cooking time: 12 minutes
Servings: 4
Ingredients:
- 4 sea bass fillets, boneless
- Sal and black pepper to the taste
- 2 cups potato chips, crushed
- 1 tablespoon mayonnaise

Directions:
1. Season the fish fillets with salt and pepper, brush with the mayonnaise and dredge each in the potato chips.
2. Arrange the fillets on a baking sheet lined with parchment paper and bake at 400 degrees F for 12 minutes.
3. Divide the fish between plates and serve with a side salad.

Nutrition: calories 228, fat 8.6, fiber 0.6, carbs 9.3, protein 25

Fish and Tomato Sauce

Preparation time: 10 minutes
Cooking time: 30 minutes
Servings: 4
Ingredients:
- 4 cod fillets, boneless
- 2 garlic cloves, minced
- 2 cups cherry tomatoes, halved
- 1 cup chicken stock
- A pinch of salt and black pepper
- ¼ cup basil, chopped

Directions:
1. Put the tomatoes, garlic, salt and pepper in a pan, heat up over medium heat and cook for 5 minutes.
2. Add the fish and the rest of the ingredients, bring to a simmer, cover the pan and cook for 25 minutes.
3. Divide the mix between plates and serve.
Nutrition: calories 180, fat 1.9, fiber 1.4, carbs 5.3, protein 33.8

Halibut and Quinoa Mix

Preparation time: 10 minutes
Cooking time: 12 minutes
Servings: 4
Ingredients:
- 4 halibut fillets, boneless
- 2 tablespoons olive oil
- 1 teaspoon rosemary, dried
- 2 teaspoons cumin, ground
- 1 tablespoons coriander, ground
- 2 teaspoons cinnamon powder
- 2 teaspoons oregano, dried
- A pinch of salt and black pepper
- 2 cups quinoa, cooked
- 1 cup cherry tomatoes, halved
- 1 avocado, peeled, pitted and sliced
- 1 cucumber, cubed
- ½ cup black olives, pitted and sliced
- Juice of 1 lemon

Directions:
1. In a bowl, combine the fish with the rosemary, cumin, coriander, cinnamon, oregano, salt and pepper and toss.
2. Heat up a pan with the oil over medium heat, add the fish, and sear for 2 minutes on each side.
3. Introduce the pan in the oven and bake the fish at 425 degrees F for 7 minutes.
4. Meanwhile, in a bowl, mix the quinoa with the remaining ingredients, toss and divide between plates.
5. Add the fish next to the quinoa mix and serve right away.
Nutrition: calories 364, fat 15.4, fiber 11.2, carbs 56.4, protein 24.5

Lemon and Dates Barramundi

Preparation time: 10 minutes
Cooking time: 12 minutes
Servings: 2
Ingredients:
- 2 barramundi fillets, boneless
- 1 shallot, sliced
- 4 lemon slices
- Juice of ½ lemon
- Zest of 1 lemon, grated
- 2 tablespoons olive oil
- 6 ounces baby spinach
- ¼ cup almonds, chopped
- 4 dates, pitted and chopped
- ¼ cup parsley, chopped
- Salt and black pepper to the taste

Directions:
1. Season the fish with salt and pepper and arrange on 2 parchment paper pieces.
2. Top the fish with the lemon slices, drizzle the lemon juice, and then top with the other ingredients except the oil.
3. Drizzle 1 tablespoon oil over each fish mix, wrap the parchment paper around the fish shaping to packets and arrange them on a baking sheet.
4. Bake at 400 degrees F for 12 minutes, cool the mix a bit, unfold, divide everything between plates and serve.

Nutrition: calories 232, fat 16.5, fiber 11.1, carbs 24.8, protein 6.5

Fish Cakes

Preparation time: 10 minutes
Cooking time: 10 minutes
Servings: 6
Ingredients:
- 20 ounces canned sardines, drained and mashed well
- 2 garlic cloves, minced
- 2 tablespoons dill, chopped
- 1 yellow onion, chopped
- 1 cup panko breadcrumbs
- 1 egg, whisked
- A pinch of salt and black pepper
- 2 tablespoons lemon juice
- 5 tablespoons olive oil

Directions:
1. In a bowl, combine the sardines with the garlic, dill and the rest of the ingredients except the oil, stir well and shape medium cakes out of this mix.
2. Heat up a pan with the oil over medium-high heat, add the fish cakes, cook for 5 minutes on each side.
3. Serve the cakes with a side salad.

Nutrition: calories 288, fat 12.8, fiber 10.2, carbs 22.2, protein 6.8

Catfish Fillets and Rice

Preparation time: 10 minutes
Cooking time: 55 minutes
Servings: 2
Ingredients:
- 2 catfish fillets, boneless
- 2 tablespoons Italian seasoning
- 2 tablespoons olive oil

For the rice:
- 1 cup brown rice
- 2 tablespoons olive oil
- 1 and ½ cups water
- ½ cup green bell pepper, chopped
- 2 garlic cloves, minced
- ½ cup white onion, chopped
- 2 teaspoons Cajun seasoning
- ½ teaspoon garlic powder
- Salt and black pepper to the taste

Directions:
1. Heat up a pot with 2 tablespoons oil over medium heat, add the onion, garlic, garlic powder, salt and pepper and sauté for 5 minutes.
2. Add the rice, water, bell pepper and the seasoning, bring to a simmer and cook over medium heat for 40 minutes.
3. Heat up a pan with 2 tablespoons oil over medium heat, add the fish and the Italian seasoning, and cook for 5 minutes on each side.
4. Divide the rice between plates, add the fish on top and serve.

Nutrition: calories 261, fat 17.6, fiber 12.2, carbs 24.8, protein 12.5

Halibut Pan

Preparation time: 10 minutes
Cooking time: 20 minutes
Servings: 4
Ingredients:
- 4 halibut fillets, boneless
- 1 red bell pepper, chopped
- 2 tablespoons olive oil
- 1 yellow onion, chopped
- 4 garlic cloves, minced
- ½ cup chicken stock
- 1 teaspoon basil, dried
- ½ cup cherry tomatoes, halved
- 1/3 cup kalamata olives, pitted and halved
- Salt and black pepper to the taste

Directions:
1. Heat up a pan with the oil over medium heat, add the fish, cook for 5 minutes on each side and divide between plates.
2. Add the onion, bell pepper, garlic and tomatoes to the pan, stir and sauté for 3 minutes.
3. Add salt, pepper and the rest of the ingredients, toss, cook for 3 minutes more, divide next to the fish and serve.

Nutrition: calories 253, fat 8, fiber 1, carbs 5, protein 28

Baked Shrimp Mix

Preparation time: 10 minutes
Cooking time: 32 minutes

Servings: 4
Ingredients:
- 4 gold potatoes, peeled and sliced
- 2 fennel bulbs, trimmed and cut into wedges
- 2 shallots, chopped
- 2 garlic cloves, minced
- 3 tablespoons olive oil
- ½ cup kalamata olives, pitted and halved
- 2 pounds shrimp, peeled and deveined
- 1 teaspoon lemon zest, grated
- 2 teaspoons oregano, dried
- 4 ounces feta cheese, crumbled
- 2 tablespoons parsley, chopped

Directions:
1.   In a roasting pan, combine the potatoes with 2 tablespoons oil, garlic and the rest of the ingredients except the shrimp, toss, introduce in the oven and bake at 450 degrees F for 25 minutes.
2.   Add the shrimp, toss, bake for 7 minutes more, divide between plates and serve.
Nutrition: calories 341, fat 19, fiber 9, carbs 34, protein 10

Shrimp and Lemon Sauce

Preparation time: 10 minutes
Cooking time: 15 minutes
Servings: 4
Ingredients:
- 1 pound shrimp, peeled and deveined
- 1/3 cup lemon juice
- 4 egg yolks
- 2 tablespoons olive oil
- 1 cup chicken stock
- Salt and black pepper to the taste
- 1 cup black olives, pitted and halved
- 1 tablespoon thyme, chopped

Directions:
1.   In a bowl, mix the lemon juice with the egg yolks and whisk well.
2.   Heat up a pan with the oil over medium heat, add the shrimp and cook for 2 minutes on each side and transfer to a plate.
3.   Heat up a pan with the stock over medium heat, add some of this over the egg yolks and lemon juice mix and whisk well.
4.   Add this over the rest of the stock, also add salt and pepper, whisk well and simmer for 2 minutes.
5.   Add the shrimp and the rest of the ingredients, toss and serve right away.
Nutrition: calories 237, fat 15.3, fiber 4.6, carbs 15.4, protein 7.6

Shrimp and Beans Salad

Preparation time: 10 minutes
Cooking time: 4 minutes
Servings: 4
Ingredients:
- 1 pound shrimp, peeled and deveined
- 30 ounces canned cannellini beans, drained and rinsed

- 2 tablespoons olive oil
- 1 cup cherry tomatoes, halved
- 1 teaspoon lemon zest, grated
- ½ cup red onion, chopped
- 4 handfuls baby arugula
- A pinch of salt and black pepper

For the dressing:
- 3 tablespoons red wine vinegar
- 2 garlic cloves, minced
- ½ cup olive oil

Directions:
1.   Heat up a pan with 2 tablespoons oil over medium-high heat, add the shrimp and cook for 2 minutes on each side.
2.   In a salad bowl, combine the shrimp with the beans and the rest of the ingredients except the ones for the dressing and toss.
3.   In a separate bowl, combine the vinegar with ½ cup oil and the garlic and whisk well.
4.   Pour over the salad, toss and serve right away.
Nutrition: calories 207, fat 12.3, fiber 6.6, carbs 15.4, protein 8.7

Pecan Salmon Fillets

Preparation time: 10 minutes
Cooking time: 15 minutes
Servings: 6
Ingredients:
- 3 tablespoons olive oil
- 3 tablespoons mustard
- 5 teaspoons honey
- 1 cup pecans, chopped
- 6 salmon fillets, boneless
- 1 tablespoon lemon juice
- 3 teaspoons parsley, chopped
- Salt and pepper to the taste

Directions:
1.   In a bowl, mix the oil with the mustard and honey and whisk well.
2.   Put the pecans and the parsley in another bowl.
3.   Season the salmon fillets with salt and pepper, arrange them on a baking sheet lined with parchment paper, brush with the honey and mustard mix and top with the pecans mix.
4.   Introduce in the oven at 400 degrees F, bake for 15 minutes, divide between plates, drizzle the lemon juice on top and serve.
Nutrition: calories 282, fat 15.5, fiber 8.5, carbs 20.9, protein 16.8

Salmon and Broccoli

Preparation time: 10 minutes
Cooking time: 20 minutes
Servings: 4
Ingredients:
- 2 tablespoons balsamic vinegar
- 1 broccoli head, florets separated
- 4 pieces salmon fillets, skinless
- 1 big red onion, roughly chopped
- 1 tablespoon olive oil

- Sea salt and black pepper to the taste

Directions:
1. In a baking dish, combine the salmon with the broccoli and the rest of the ingredients, introduce in the oven and bake at 390 degrees F for 20 minutes.
2. Divide the mix between plates and serve.

Nutrition: calories 302, fat 15.5, fiber 8.5, carbs 18.9, protein 19.8

Salmon and Peach Pan

Preparation time: 10 minutes
Cooking time: 11 minutes
Servings: 4
Ingredients:
- 1 tablespoon balsamic vinegar
- 1 teaspoon thyme, chopped
- 1 tablespoon ginger, grated
- 2 tablespoons olive oil
- Sea salt and black pepper to the taste
- 3 peaches, cut into medium wedges
- 4 salmon fillets, boneless

Directions:
1. Heat up a pan with the oil over medium-high heat, add the salmon and cook for 3 minutes on each side.
2. Add the vinegar, the peaches and the rest of the ingredients, cook for 5 minutes more, divide everything between plates and serve.

Nutrition: calories 293, fat 17.1, fiber 4.1, carbs 26.4, protein 24.5

Tarragon Cod Fillets

Preparation time: 10 minutes
Cooking time: 12 minutes
Servings: 4
Ingredients:
- 4 cod fillets, boneless
- ¼ cup capers, drained
- 1 tablespoon tarragon, chopped
- Sea salt and black pepper to the taste
- 2 tablespoons olive oil
- 2 tablespoons parsley, chopped
- 1 tablespoon olive oil
- 1 tablespoon lemon juice

Directions:
1. Heat up a pan with the oil over medium-high heat, add the fish and cook for 3 minutes on each side.
2. Add the rest of the ingredients, cook everything for 7 minutes more, divide between plates and serve.

Nutrition: calories 162, fat 9.6, fiber 4.3, carbs 12.4, protein 16.5

Salmon and Radish Mix

Preparation time: 10 minutes
Cooking time: 15 minutes
Servings: 4
Ingredients:
- 2 tablespoons olive oil
- 1 tablespoon balsamic vinegar
- 1 and ½ cup chicken stock

- 4 salmon fillets, boneless
- 2 garlic cloves, minced
- 1 tablespoon ginger, grated
- 1 cup radishes, grated
- ¼ cup scallions, chopped

Directions:
1. Heat up a pan with the oil over medium-high heat, add the salmon, cook for 4 minutes on each side and divide between plates
2. Add the vinegar and the rest of the ingredients to the pan, toss gently, cook for 10 minutes, add over the salmon and serve.

Nutrition: calories 274, fat 14.5, fiber 3.5, carbs 8.5, protein 22.3

Smoked Salmon and Watercress Salad

Preparation time: 5 minutes
Cooking time: 0 minutes
Servings: 4
Ingredients:
- 2 bunches watercress
- 1 pound smoked salmon, skinless, boneless and flaked
- 2 teaspoons mustard
- ¼ cup lemon juice
- ½ cup Greek yogurt
- Salt and black pepper to the taste
- 1 big cucumber, sliced
- 2 tablespoons chives, chopped

Directions:
1. In a salad bowl, combine the salmon with the watercress and the rest of the ingredients toss and serve right away.

Nutrition: calories 244, fat 16.7, fiber 4.5, carbs 22.5, protein 15.6

Salmon and Corn Salad

Preparation time: 5 minutes
Cooking time: 0 minutes
Servings: 4
Ingredients:
- ½ cup pecans, chopped
- 2 cups baby arugula
- 1 cup corn
- ¼ pound smoked salmon, skinless, boneless and cut into small chunks
- 2 tablespoons olive oil
- 2 tablespoon lemon juice
- Sea salt and black pepper to the taste

Directions:
1. In a salad bowl, combine the salmon with the corn and the rest of the ingredients, toss and serve right away.

Nutrition: calories 284, fat 18.4, fiber 5.4, carbs 22.6, protein 17.4

Cod and Mushrooms Mix

Preparation time: 10 minutes
Cooking time: 25 minutes

Servings: 4
Ingredients:
- 2 cod fillets, boneless
- 4 tablespoons olive oil
- 4 ounces mushrooms, sliced
- Sea salt and black pepper to the taste
- 12 cherry tomatoes, halved
- 8 ounces lettuce leaves, torn
- 1 avocado, pitted, peeled and cubed
- 1 red chili pepper, chopped
- 1 tablespoon cilantro, chopped
- 2 tablespoons balsamic vinegar
- 1 ounce feta cheese, crumbled

Directions:
1.   Put the fish in a roasting pan, brush it with 2 tablespoons oil, sprinkle salt and pepper all over and broil under medium-high heat for 15 minutes. Meanwhile, heat up a pan with the rest of the oil over medium heat, add the mushrooms, stir and sauté for 5 minutes.
2.   Add the rest of the ingredients, toss, cook for 5 minutes more and divide between plates.
3.   Top with the fish and serve right away.
Nutrition: calories 257, fat 10, fiber 3.1, carbs 24.3, protein 19.4

Sesame Shrimp Mix

Preparation time: 10 minutes
Cooking time: 0 minutes
Servings: 4
Ingredients:
- 2 tablespoon lime juice
- 3 tablespoons teriyaki sauce
- 2 tablespoons olive oil
- 8 cups baby spinach
- 14 ounces shrimp, cooked, peeled and deveined
- 1 cup cucumber, sliced
- 1 cup radish, sliced
- ¼ cup cilantro, chopped
- 2 teaspoons sesame seeds, toasted

Directions:
1.   In a bowl, mix the shrimp with the lime juice, spinach and the rest of the ingredients, toss and serve cold.
Nutrition: calories 177, fat 9, fiber 7.1, carbs 14.3, protein 9.4

Creamy Curry Salmon

Preparation time: 10 minutes
Cooking time: 20 minutes
Servings: 2
Ingredients:
- 2 salmon fillets, boneless and cubed
- 1 tablespoon olive oil
- 1 tablespoon basil, chopped
- Sea salt and black pepper to the taste
- 1 cup Greek yogurt
- 2 teaspoons curry powder
- 1 garlic clove, minced
- ½ teaspoon mint, chopped

Directions:
1.   Heat up a pan with the oil over medium-high heat, add the salmon and cook for 3 minutes.
2.   Add the rest of the ingredients, toss, cook for 15 minutes more, divide between plates and serve.
Nutrition: calories 284, fat 14.1, fiber 8.5, carbs 26.7, protein 31.4

Mahi Mahi and Pomegranate Sauce

Preparation time: 10 minutes
Cooking time: 10 minutes
Servings: 4
Ingredients:
- 1 and ½ cups chicken stock
- 1 tablespoon olive oil
- 4 mahi mahi fillets, boneless
- 4 tablespoons tahini paste
- Juice of 1 lime
- Seeds from 1 pomegranate
- 1 tablespoon parsley, chopped

Directions:
1.   Heat up a pan with the oil over medium-high heat, add the fish and cook for 3 minutes on each side.
2.   Add the rest of the ingredients, flip the fish again, cook for 4 minutes more, divide everything between plates and serve.
Nutrition: calories 224, fat 11.1, fiber 5.5, carbs 16.7, protein 11.4

Smoked Salmon and Veggies Mix

Preparation time: 10 minutes
Cooking time: 20 minutes
Servings: 4
Ingredients:
- 3 red onions, cut into wedges
- ¾ cup green olives, pitted and halved
- 3 red bell peppers, roughly chopped
- ½ teaspoon smoked paprika
- Salt and black pepper to the taste
- 3 tablespoons olive oil
- 4 salmon fillets, skinless and boneless
- 2 tablespoons chives, chopped

Directions:
1.   In a roasting pan, combine the salmon with the onions and the rest of the ingredients, introduce in the oven and bake at 390 degrees F for 20 minutes.
2.   Divide the mix between plates and serve.
Nutrition: calories 301, fat 5.9, fiber 11.9, carbs 26.4, protein 22.4

Salmon and Mango Mix

Preparation time: 10 minutes
Cooking time: 25 minutes
Servings: 2
Ingredients:
- 2 salmon fillets, skinless and boneless
- Salt and pepper to the taste
- 2 tablespoons olive oil
- 2 garlic cloves, minced
- 2 mangos, peeled and cubed

- 1 red chili, chopped
- 1 small piece ginger, grated
- Juice of 1 lime
- 1 tablespoon cilantro, chopped

Directions:

1. In a roasting pan, combine the salmon with the oil, garlic and the rest of the ingredients except the cilantro, toss, introduce in the oven at 350 degrees F and bake for 25 minutes.
2. Divide everything between plates and serve with the cilantro sprinkled on top.

Nutrition: calories 251, fat 15.9, fiber 5.9, carbs 26.4, protein 12.4

Salmon and Creamy Endives

Preparation time: 10 minutes
Cooking time: 15 minutes
Servings: 4
Ingredients:

- 4 salmon fillets, boneless
- 2 endives, shredded
- Juice of 1 lime
- Salt and black pepper to the taste
- ¼ cup chicken stock
- 1 cup Greek yogurt
- ¼ cup green olives pitted and chopped
- ¼ cup fresh chives, chopped
- 3 tablespoons olive oil

Directions:

1. Heat up a pan with half of the oil over medium heat, add the endives and the rest of the ingredients except the chives and the salmon, toss, cook for 6 minutes and divide between plates.
2. Heat up another pan with the rest of the oil, add the salmon, season with salt and pepper, cook for 4 minutes on each side, add next to the creamy endives mix, sprinkle the chives on top and serve.

Nutrition: calories 266, fat 13.9, fiber 11.1, carbs 23.8, protein 17.5

Trout and Tzatziki Sauce

Preparation time: 10 minutes
Cooking time: 10 minutes
Servings: 4
Ingredients:

- Juice of ½ lime
- Salt and black pepper to the taste
- 1 and ½ teaspoon coriander, ground
- 1 teaspoon garlic, minced
- 4 trout fillets, boneless
- 1 teaspoon sweet paprika
- 2 tablespoons avocado oil

For the sauce:

- 1 cucumber, chopped
- 4 garlic cloves, minced
- 1 tablespoon olive oil
- 1 teaspoon white vinegar
- 1 and ½ cups Greek yogurt
- A pinch of salt and white pepper

Directions:

1. Heat up a pan with the avocado oil over medium-high heat, add the fish, salt, pepper, lime juice, 1 teaspoon garlic and the paprika, rub the fish gently and cook for 4 minutes on each side.
2. In a bowl, combine the cucumber with 4 garlic cloves and the rest of the ingredients for the sauce and whisk well.
3. Divide the fish between plates, drizzle the sauce all over and serve with a side salad.

Nutrition: calories 393, fat 18.5, fiber 6.5, carbs 18.3, protein 39.6

Parsley Trout and Capers

Preparation time: 10 minutes
Cooking time: 10 minutes
Servings: 4
Ingredients:

- 4 trout fillets, boneless
- 3 ounces tomato sauce
- A handful parsley, chopped
- 2 tablespoons olive oil
- Salt and black pepper to the taste

Directions:

1. Heat up a pan with the oil over medium-high heat, add the fish, salt and pepper and cook for 3 minutes on each side.
2. Add the rest of the ingredients, cook everything for 4 minutes more.
3. Divide everything between plates and serve.

Nutrition: calories 308, fat 17, fiber 1, carbs 3, protein 16

Baked Trout and Fennel

Preparation time: 10 minutes
Cooking time: 22 minutes
Servings: 4
Ingredients:

- 1 fennel bulb, sliced
- 2 tablespoons olive oil
- 1 yellow onion, sliced
- 3 teaspoons Italian seasoning
- 4 rainbow trout fillets, boneless
- ¼ cup panko breadcrumbs
- ½ cup kalamata olives, pitted and halved
- Juice of 1 lemon

Directions:

1. Spread the fennel the onion and the rest of the ingredients except the trout and the breadcrumbs on a baking sheet lined with parchment paper, toss them and cook at 400 degrees F for 10 minutes.
2. Add the fish dredged in breadcrumbs and seasoned with salt and pepper and cook it at 400 degrees F for 6 minutes on each side.
3. Divide the mix between plates and serve.

Nutrition: calories 306, fat 8.9, fiber 11.1, carbs 23.8, protein 14.5

Lemon Rainbow Trout

Preparation time: 10 minutes
Cooking time: 15 minutes
Servings: 2

Ingredients:
- 2 rainbow trout
- Juice of 1 lemon
- 3 tablespoons olive oil
- 4 garlic cloves, minced
- A pinch of salt and black pepper

Directions:
1. Line a baking sheet with parchment paper, add the fish and the rest of the ingredients and rub.
2. Bake at 400 degrees F for 15 minutes, divide between plates and serve with a side salad.

Nutrition: calories 521, fat 29, fiber 5, carbs 14, protein 52

Trout and Peppers Mix

Preparation time: 10 minutes
Cooking time: 20 minutes
Servings: 4
Ingredients:
- 4 trout fillets, boneless
- 2 tablespoons kalamata olives, pitted and chopped
- 1 tablespoon capers, drained
- 2 tablespoons olive oil
- A pinch of salt and black pepper
- 1 and ½ teaspoons chili powder
- 1 yellow bell pepper, chopped
- 1 red bell pepper, chopped
- 1 green bell pepper, chopped

Directions:
1. Heat up a pan with the oil over medium-high heat, add the trout, salt and pepper and cook for 10 minutes.
2. Flip the fish, add the peppers and the rest of the ingredients, cook for 10 minutes more, divide the whole mix between plates and serve.

Nutrition: calories 572, fat 17.4, fiber 6, carbs 71, protein 33.7

Cod and Cabbage

Preparation time: 10 minutes
Cooking time: 15 minutes
Servings: 4
Ingredients:
- 3 cups green cabbage, shredded
- 1 sweet onion, sliced
- A pinch of salt and black pepper
- ½ cup feta cheese, crumbled
- 4 teaspoons olive oil
- 4 cod fillets, boneless
- ¼ cup green olives, pitted and chopped

Directions:
1. Grease a roasting pan with the oil, add the fish, the cabbage and the rest of the ingredients, introduce in the pan and cook at 450 degrees F for 15 minutes.
2. Divide the mix between plates and serve.

Nutrition: calories 270, fat 10, fiber 3, carbs 12, protein 31

Mediterranean Mussels

Preparation time: 10 minutes
Cooking time: 10 minutes
Servings: 4
Ingredients:
- 1 white onion, sliced
- 3 tablespoons olive oil
- 2 teaspoons fennel seeds
- 4 garlic cloves, minced
- 1 teaspoon red pepper, crushed
- A pinch of salt and black pepper
- 1 cup chicken stock
- 1 tablespoon lemon juice
- 2 and ½ pounds mussels, scrubbed
- ½ cup parsley, chopped
- ½ cup tomatoes, cubed

Directions:
1. Heat up a pan with the oil over medium-high heat, add the onion and the garlic and sauté for 2 minutes.
2. Add the rest of the ingredients except the mussels, stir and cook for 3 minutes more.
3. Add the mussels, cook everything for 6 minutes more, divide everything into bowls and serve.

Nutrition: calories 276, fat 9.8, fiber 4.8, carbs 6.5, protein 20.5

Mussels Bowls

Preparation time: 10 minutes
Cooking time: 10 minutes
Servings: 4
Ingredients:
- 2 pounds mussels, scrubbed
- 1 tablespoon garlic, minced
- 1 tablespoon basil, chopped
- 1 yellow onion, chopped
- 6 tomatoes, cubed
- 1 cup heavy cream
- 2 tablespoons olive oil
- 1 tablespoon parsley, chopped

Directions:
1. Heat up a pan with the oil over medium-high heat, add the garlic and the onion and sauté for 2 minutes.
2. Add the mussels and the rest of the ingredients, toss, cook for 7 minutes more, divide into bowls and serve.

Nutrition: calories 266, fat 11.8, fiber 5.8, carbs 16.5, protein 10.5

Calamari and Dill Sauce

Preparation time: 10 minutes
Cooking time: 15 minutes
Servings: 4
Ingredients:
- 1 and ½ pound calamari, sliced into rings
- 10 garlic cloves, minced
- 2 tablespoons olive oil
- Juice of 1 and ½ lime
- 2 tablespoons balsamic vinegar

- 3 tablespoons dill, chopped
- A pinch of salt and black pepper

Directions:
1. Heat up a pan with the oil over medium-high heat, add the garlic, lime juice and the other ingredients except the calamari and cook for 5 minutes.
2. Add the calamari rings, cook everything for 10 minutes more, divide between plates and serve.

Nutrition: calories 282, fat 18.6, fiber 4, carbs 9.2, protein 18.5

Chili Calamari and Veggie Mix

Preparation time: 10 minutes
Cooking time: 40 minutes
Servings: 4
Ingredients:
- 1 pound calamari rings
- 2 red chili peppers, chopped
- 2 tablespoons olive oil
- 3 garlic cloves, minced
- 14 ounces canned tomatoes, chopped
- 2 tablespoons tomato paste
- 1 tablespoon thyme, chopped
- Salt and black pepper to the taste
- 2 tablespoons capers, drained
- 12 black olives, pitted and halved

Directions:
1. Heat up a pan with the oil over medium-high heat, add the garlic and the chili peppers and sauté for 2 minutes.
2. Add the rest of the ingredients except the olives and capers, stir, bring to a simmer and cook for 22 minutes.
3. Add the olives and capers, cook everything for 15 minutes more, divide everything into bowls and serve.

Nutrition: calories 274, fat 11.6, fiber 2.8, carbs 13.5, protein 15.4

Cheesy Crab and Lime Spread

Preparation time: 10 minutes
Cooking time: 25 minutes
Servings: 8
Ingredients:
- 1 pound crab meat, flaked
- 4 ounces cream cheese, soft
- 1 tablespoon chives, chopped
- 1 teaspoon lime juice
- 1 teaspoon lime zest, grated

Directions:
1. In a baking dish greased with cooking spray, combine the crab with the rest of the ingredients and toss.
2. Introduce in the oven at 350 degrees F, bake for 25 minutes, divide into bowls and serve.

Nutrition: calories 284, fat 14.6, fiber 5.8, carbs 16.5, protein 15.4

Horseradish Cheesy Salmon Mix

Preparation time: 1 hour
Cooking time: 0 minutes
Servings: 8
Ingredients:
- 2 ounces feta cheese, crumbled
- 4 ounces cream cheese, soft
- 3 tablespoons already prepared horseradish
- 1 pound smoked salmon, skinless, boneless and flaked
- 2 teaspoons lime zest, grated
- 1 red onion, chopped
- 3 tablespoons chives, chopped

Directions:
1. In your food processor, mix cream cheese with horseradish, goat cheese and lime zest and blend very well.
2. In a bowl, combine the salmon with the rest of the ingredients, toss and serve cold.

Nutrition: calories 281, fat 17.9, fiber 1, carbs 4.2, protein 25.3

Greek Trout Spread

Preparation time: 5 minutes
Cooking time: 0 minutes
Servings: 8
Ingredients:
- 4 ounces smoked trout, skinless, boneless and flaked
- 1 tablespoon lemon juice
- 1 cup Greek yogurt
- tablespoon dill, chopped
- Salt and black pepper to the taste
- A drizzle of olive oil

Directions:
1. In a bowl, combine the trout with the lemon juice and the rest of the ingredients and whisk really well.
2. Divide the spread into bowls and serve.

Nutrition: calories 258, fat 4,5, fiber 2, carbs 5.5, protein 7.6

Scallions and Salmon Tartar

Preparation time: 5 minutes
Cooking time: 0 minutes
Servings: 4
Ingredients:
- 4 tablespoons scallions, chopped
- 2 teaspoons lemon juice
- 1 tablespoon chives, minced
- 1 tablespoon olive oil
- 1 pound salmon, skinless, boneless and minced
- Salt and black pepper to the taste
- 1 tablespoon parsley, chopped

Directions:
1. In a bowl, combine the scallions with the salmon and the rest of the ingredients, stir well, divide into small moulds between plates and serve.

Nutrition: calories 224, fat 14.5, fiber 5.2, carbs 12.7, protein 5.3

Salmon and Green Beans

Preparation time: 10 minutes
Cooking time: 15 minutes
Servings: 4
Ingredients:
- 3 tablespoons balsamic vinegar
- 2 tablespoons olive oil
- 1 garlic clove, minced
- ½ teaspoons red pepper flakes, crushed
- ½ teaspoon lime zest, grated
- 1 and ½ pounds green beans, chopped
- Salt and black pepper to the taste
- 1 red onion, sliced
- 4 salmon fillets, boneless

Directions:
1. Heat up a pan with half of the oil, add the vinegar, onion, garlic and the other ingredients except the salmon, toss, cook for 6 minutes and divide between plates.
2. Heat up the same pan with the rest of the oil over medium-high heat, add the salmon, salt and pepper, cook for 4 minutes on each side, add next to the green beans and serve.

Nutrition: calories 224, fat 15.5, fiber 8.2, carbs 22.7, protein 16.3

Cayenne Cod and Tomatoes

Preparation time: 10 minutes
Cooking time: 25 minutes
Servings: 4
Ingredients:
- 1 teaspoon lime juice
- Salt and black pepper to the taste
- 1 teaspoon sweet paprika
- 1 teaspoon cayenne pepper
- 2 tablespoons olive oil
- 1 yellow onion, chopped
- 2 garlic cloves, minced
- 4 cod fillets, boneless
- A pinch of cloves, ground
- ½ cup chicken stock
- ½ pound cherry tomatoes, cubed

Directions:
1. Heat up a pan with the oil over medium-high heat add the cod, salt, pepper and the cayenne, cook for 4 minutes on each side and divide between plates.
2. Heat up the same pan over medium-high heat, add the onion and garlic and sauté for 5 minutes.
3. Add the rest of the ingredients, stir, bring to a simmer and cook for 10 minutes more.
4. Divide the mix next to the fish and serve.

Nutrition: calories 232, fat 16.5, fiber 11.1, carbs 24.8, protein 16.5

Salmon and Watermelon Gazpacho

Preparation time: 4 hours
Cooking time: 0 minutes
Servings: 4
Ingredients:
- ¼ cup basil, chopped
- 1 pound tomatoes, cubed
- 1 pound watermelon, cubed
- ¼ cup red wine vinegar
- 1/3 cup avocado oil
- 2 garlic cloves, minced
- 1 cup smoked salmon, skinless, boneless and cubed
- A pinch of salt and black pepper

Directions:
1. In your blender, combine the basil with the watermelon and the rest of the ingredients except the salmon, pulse well and divide into bowls.
2. Top each serving with the salmon and serve cold.

Nutrition: calories 252, fat 16.5, fiber 9.1, carbs 24.8, protein 15.5

Shrimp and Calamari Mix

Preparation time: 10 minutes
Cooking time: 12 minutes
Servings: 4
Ingredients:
- 1 pound shrimp, peeled and deveined
- Salt and black pepper to the taste
- 3 garlic cloves, minced
- 1 tablespoon avocado oil
- ½ pound calamari rings
- ½ teaspoon basil, dried
- 1 teaspoon rosemary, dried
- 1 red onion, chopped
- 1 cup chicken stock
- Juice of 1 lemon
- 1 tablespoon parsley, chopped

Directions:
1. Heat up a pan with the oil over medium-high heat, add the onion and the garlic and sauté for 4 minutes.
2. Add the shrimp, the calamari and the rest of the ingredients except the parsley, stir, bring to a simmer and cook for 8 minutes.
3. Add the parsley, divide everything into bowls and serve.

Nutrition: calories 288, fat 12.8, fiber 10.2, carbs 22.2, protein 6.8

Shrimp and Dill Mix

Preparation time: 10 minutes
Cooking time: 10 minutes
Servings: 4
Ingredients:
- 1 pound shrimp, cooked, peeled and deveined
- ½ cup raisins
- 1 cup spring onion, chopped
- 2 tablespoons olive oil
- 2 tablespoons capers, chopped
- 2 tablespoons dill, chopped
- Salt and black pepper to the taste

Directions:

1.	Heat up a pan with the oil over medium-high heat, add the onions and raisins and sauté for 2-3 minutes.
2.	Add the shrimp and the rest of the ingredients, toss, cook for 6 minutes more, divide between plates and serve with a side salad.
Nutrition: calories 218, fat 12.8, fiber 6.2, carbs 22.2, protein 4.8

Minty Sardines Salad

Preparation time: 10 minutes
Cooking time: 0 minutes
Servings: 4
Ingredients:
•	4 ounces canned sardines in olive oil, skinless, boneless and flaked
•	2 teaspoons avocado oil
•	2 tablespoons mint, chopped
•	A pinch of salt and black pepper
•	1 avocado, peeled, pitted and cubed
•	1 cucumber, cubed
•	2 tomatoes, cubed
•	2 spring onions, chopped
Directions:
1.	In a bowl, combine the sardines with the oil and the rest of the ingredients, toss, divide into small cups and keep in the fridge for 10 minutes before serving.
Nutrition: calories 261, fat 7.6, fiber 2.2, carbs 22.8, protein 12.5

Salmon and Zucchini Rolls

Preparation time: 10 minutes
Cooking time: 0 minutes
Servings: 8
Ingredients:
•	8 slices smoked salmon, boneless
•	2 zucchinis, sliced lengthwise in 8 pieces
•	1 cup ricotta cheese, soft
•	2 teaspoons lemon zest, grated
•	1 tablespoon dill, chopped
•	1 small red onion, sliced
•	Salt and pepper to the taste
Directions:
1.	In a bowl, mix the ricotta cheese with the rest of the ingredients except the salmon and the zucchini and whisk well.
2.	Arrange the zucchini slices on a working surface, and divide the salmon on top.
3.	Spread the cheese mix all over, roll and secure with toothpicks and serve right away.
Nutrition: calories 297, fat 24.3, fiber 11.6, carbs 15.4, protein 11.6

Wrapped Scallops

Preparation time: 10 minutes
Cooking time: 6 minutes
Servings: 12
Ingredients:
•	12 medium scallops

•	12 thin bacon slices
•	2 teaspoons lemon juice
•	2 teaspoons olive oil
•	A pinch of chili powder
•	A pinch of cloves, ground
•	Salt and black pepper to the taste
Directions:
1.	Wrap each scallop in a bacon slice and secure with toothpicks.
2.	Heat up a pan with the oil over medium-high heat, add the scallops and the rest of the ingredients, cook for 3 minutes on each side, divide between plates and serve.
Nutrition: calories 297, fat 24.3, fiber 9.6, carbs 22.4, protein 17.6

Chorizo Shrimp and Salmon Mix

Preparation time: 10 minutes
Cooking time: 20 minutes
Servings: 4
Ingredients:
•	3 tablespoons olive oil
•	1 pound shrimp, peeled and deveined
•	1 pound salmon, skinless, boneless and cubed
•	4 ounces chorizo, chopped
•	Salt and black pepper to the taste
•	3 cups canned tomatoes, crushed
•	1 red onion, chopped
•	2 garlic cloves, minced
•	¼ teaspoon red pepper flakes, crushed
•	1 cup chicken stock
•	1 tablespoon cilantro, chopped
Directions:
1.	Heat up a pan with the olive oil over medium-high heat, add the chorizo and cook for 2 minutes.
2.	Add salt, pepper, tomatoes, and the rest of the ingredients except the shrimp, salmon and the cilantro, stir, bring to a simmer and cook for 10 minutes.
3.	Add the remaining ingredients, cook everything for 8 minutes more, divide into bowls and serve.
Nutrition: calories 232, fat 15.5, fiber 10.5, carbs 20.9, protein 16.8

Garlic Scallops and Peas Mix

Preparation time: 10 minutes
Cooking time: 20 minutes
Servings: 6
Ingredients:
•	12 ounces scallops
•	2 tablespoons olive oil
•	4 garlic cloves, minced
•	A pinch of salt and black pepper
•	½ cup chicken stock
•	1 cup snow peas, sliced
•	½ tablespoon balsamic vinegar
•	1 cup scallions, sliced
•	1 tablespoon basil, chopped
Directions:

1. Heat up a pan with half of the oil over medium-high heat, add the scallops, cook for 5 minutes on each side and transfer to a bowl.
2. Heat up the pan again with the rest of the oil over medium heat, add the scallions and the garlic and sauté for 2 minutes.
3. Add the rest of the ingredients, stir, bring to a simmer and cook for 5 minutes more.
4. Add the scallops to the pan, cook everything for 3 minutes, divide into bowls and serve.
Nutrition: calories 296, fat 11.8, fiber 9.8, carbs 26.5, protein 20.5

Kale, Beets and Cod Mix
Preparation time: 10 minutes
Cooking time: 20 minutes
Servings: 4
Ingredients:
- 2 tablespoons apple cider vinegar
- ½ cup chicken stock
- 1 red onion, sliced
- 4 golden beets, trimmed, peeled and cubed
- 2 tablespoons olive oil
- Salt and black pepper to the taste
- 4 cups kale, torn
- 2 tablespoons walnuts, chopped
- 1 pound cod fillets, boneless, skinless and cubed

Directions:
1. Heat up a pan with the oil over medium-high heat, add the onion and the beets and cook for 3-4 minutes.
2. Add the rest of the ingredients except the fish and the walnuts, stir, bring to a simmer and cook for 5 minutes more.
3. Add the fish, cook for 10 minutes, divide between plates and serve.
Nutrition: calories 285, fat 7.6, fiber 6.5, carbs 16.7, protein 12.5

Salmon, Calamari And Mango Mix
Preparation time: 10 minutes
Cooking time: 10 minutes
Servings: 4
Ingredients:
- ½ pound smoked salmon, skinless, boneless and cubed
- ½ pound calamari rings
- 1 tablespoon garlic chili sauce
- 2 tablespoons olive oil
- ¼ cup lime juice
- ½ teaspoon smoked paprika
- ½ teaspoon cumin, ground
- 2 garlic cloves, minced
- A pinch of salt and black pepper
- 1 cup mango, peeled and cubed

Directions:
1. Heat up a pan with the oil over medium-high heat, add the garlic sauce, lime juice and the rest of the ingredients except the salmon and the calamari, stir and simmer for 3 minutes.
2. Add the remaining ingredients, cook everything for 7 minutes, divide into bowls and serve.
Nutrition: calories 274, fat 11.6, fiber 2.8, carbs 11.5, protein 15.4

Squid and Cucumber Mix
Preparation time: 10 minutes
Cooking time: 15 minutes
Servings: 4
Ingredients:
- 10 ounces squid, cut in medium pieces
- 2 cucumbers, chopped
- 2 tablespoons cilantro, chopped
- 1 hot jalapeno pepper, chopped
- 3 tablespoons balsamic vinegar
- 2 tablespoons olive oil
- A pinch of salt and black pepper
- 1 tablespoon dill, chopped

Directions:
1. Heat up a pan with the oil over medium-high heat, add the squid and cook for 5 minutes.
2. Add the cucumbers and the rest of the ingredients, stir, cook for 10 minutes more, divide everything between plates and serve.
Nutrition: calories 224, fat 14.5, fiber 11.2, carbs 22.7, protein 11.3

Octopus and Radish Salad
Preparation time: 2 hours
Cooking time: 1 hour and 30 minutes
Servings: 4
Ingredients:
- 1 big octopus, cleaned and tentacles separated
- 2 ounces calamari rings
- 3 garlic cloves, minced
- 1 white onion, chopped
- ¾ cup chicken stock
- 2 cups radicchio, sliced
- 2 cups radish, sliced
- 1 cup parsley, chopped
- 1 tablespoons olive oil
- Salt and black pepper to the taste

Directions:
1. Put the octopus tentacles in a pot, add the stock, add the calamari rings, salt and pepper, bring to a simmer and cook over medium heat for 1 hour and 30 minutes.
2. Drain everything, cut the tentacles into pieces and transfer them with the calamari rings to a bowl.
3. Add the rest of the ingredients, toss and keep the salad in the fridge for 2 hours before serving.
Nutrition: calories 287, fat 9.9, fiber 5.6, carbs 22, protein 8.4

Shrimp and Mushrooms Mix
Preparation time: 10 minutes
Cooking time: 12 minutes
Servings: 4

Ingredients:
- 1 pound shrimp, peeled and deveined
- 2 green onions, sliced
- ½ pound white mushrooms, sliced
- 2 tablespoons balsamic vinegar
- 2 tablespoons sesame seeds, toasted
- 2 teaspoons ginger, minced
- 2 teaspoons garlic, minced
- 3 tablespoons olive oil
- 2 tablespoons dill, chopped

Directions:
1. Heat up a pan with the oil over medium-high heat, add the green onions and the garlic and sauté for 2 minutes.
2. Add the rest of the ingredients except the shrimp and cook for 6 minutes more.
3. Add the shrimp, cook for 4 minutes, divide everything between plates and serve.

Nutrition: calories 245, fat 8.5, fiber 45.8, carbs 11.8, protein 17.7

Scallops and Carrots Mix

Preparation time: 10 minutes
Cooking time: 15 minutes
Servings: 4
Ingredients:
- 1 pound sea scallops, halved
- 2 celery stalks, sliced
- 2 tablespoons olive oil
- 3 garlic cloves, minced
- Salt and black pepper to the taste
- Juice of 1 lime
- 4 ounces baby carrots, trimmed
- 1 tablespoon capers, chopped
- 1 tablespoon mayonnaise
- 1 tablespoon rosemary, chopped
- 1 cup chicken stock

Directions:
1. Heat up a pan with the oil over medium-high heat, add the celery and the garlic and sauté for 2 minutes.
2. Add the carrots and the rest of the ingredients except the scallops and the mayonnaise, stir, bring to a simmer and cook over medium heat for 8 minutes.
3. Add the scallops and the mayo, toss, cook for 5 minutes, divide everything into bowls and serve.

Nutrition: calories 305, fat 14.5, fiber 5.8, carbs 31.8, protein 7.7

Lime Squid and Capers Mix

Preparation time: 10 minutes
Cooking time: 20 minutes
Servings: 6
Ingredients:
- 1 pound baby squid, cleaned, body and tentacles chopped
- ½ teaspoon lime zest, grated
- 1 tablespoon lime juice
- ½ teaspoon orange zest, grated
- 3 tablespoons olive oil
- 1 teaspoon red pepper flakes, crushed
- 1 tablespoon parsley, chopped
- 4 garlic cloves, minced
- 1 shallot, chopped
- 2 tablespoons capers, drained
- 1 cup chicken stock
- 2 tablespoons red wine vinegar
- Salt and black pepper to the taste

Directions:
1. Heat up a pan with the oil over medium-high heat, add the lime zest, lime juice, orange zest and the rest of the ingredients except the squid and the parsley, stir, bring to a simmer and cook over medium heat for 10 minutes.
2. Add the remaining ingredients, stir, cook everything for 10 minutes more, divide into bowls and serve.

Nutrition: calories 302, fat 8.5, fiber 9.8, carbs 21.8, protein 11.3

Leeks and Calamari Mix

Preparation time: 10 minutes
Cooking time: 15 minutes
Servings: 6
Ingredients:
- 2 tablespoon avocado oil
- 2 leeks, chopped
- 1 red onion, chopped
- Salt and black to the taste
- 1 pound calamari rings
- 1 tablespoon parsley, chopped
- 1 tablespoon chives, chopped
- 2 tablespoons tomato paste

Directions:
4. Heat up a pan with the avocado oil over medium heat, add the leeks and the onion, stir and sauté for 5 minutes.
5. Add the rest of the ingredients, toss, simmer over medium heat for 10 minutes, divide into bowls and serve.

Nutrition: calories 238, fat 9, fiber 5.6, carbs 14.4, protein 8.4

Cod and Brussels Sprouts

Preparation time: 10 minutes
Cooking time: 20 minutes
Servings: 4
Ingredients:
- 1 teaspoon garlic powder
- 1 teaspoon smoked paprika
- 2 tablespoons olive oil
- 2 pounds Brussels sprouts, trimmed and halved
- 4 cod fillets, boneless
- ½ cup tomato sauce
- 1 teaspoon Italian seasoning
- 1 tablespoon chives, chopped

Directions:
1. In a roasting pan, combine the sprouts with the garlic powder and the other ingredients except the cod and toss.

2. Put the cod on top, cover the pan with tin foil and bake at 450 degrees F for 20 minutes.
3. Divide the mix between plates and serve.
Nutrition: calories 188, fat 12.8, fiber 9.2, carbs 22.2, protein 16.8

Tarragon Trout and Beets

Preparation time: 10 minutes
Cooking time: 35 minutes
Servings: 4
Ingredients:
- 1 pound medium beets, peeled and cubed
- 3 tablespoons olive oil
- 4 trout fillets, boneless
- Salt and black pepper to the taste
- 1 tablespoon chives, chopped
- 1 tablespoon tarragon, chopped
- 3 tablespoon spring onions, chopped
- 2 tablespoons lemon juice
- ½ cup chicken stock

Directions:
1. Spread the beets on a baking sheet lined with parchment paper, add salt, pepper and 1 tablespoon oil, toss and bake at 450 degrees F for 20 minutes.
2. Heat up a pan with the rest of the oil over medium-high heat, add the trout and the remaining ingredients, and cook for 4 minutes on each side.
3. Add the baked beets, cook the mix for 5 minutes more, divide everything between plates and serve.
Nutrition: calories 232, fat 5.5, fiber 7.5, carbs 20.9, protein 16.8

Ginger Trout and Eggplant

Preparation time: 10 minutes
Cooking time: 22 minutes
Servings: 4
Ingredients:
- 4 trout fillets, boneless
- 1 eggplant, sliced
- ¼ cup tomato sauce
- 2 tablespoons olive oil
- Salt and black pepper to the taste
- 2 teaspoons ginger, grated
- 2 tablespoons balsamic vinegar
- 2 tablespoons chives, chopped

Directions:
1. Heat up a pan with the oil over medium heat, add the eggplant and the rest of the ingredients except the trout and cook for 10 minutes.
2. Add the fish on top, introduce the pan in the oven and bake at 450 degrees F for 12 minutes.
3. Divide everything between plates and serve.
Nutrition: calories 282, fat 11.5, fiber 5.5, carbs 17.9, protein 14.8

Poultry Recipes

Chicken and Olives

Preparation time: 10 minutes
Cooking time: 15 minutes
Servings: 4
Ingredients:

- 4 chicken breasts, skinless and boneless
- 2 tablespoons garlic, minced
- 1 tablespoon oregano, dried
- Salt and black pepper to the taste
- 2 tablespoons olive oil
- ½ cup chicken stock
- Juice of 1 lemon
- 1 cup red onion, chopped
- 1 and ½ cups tomatoes, cubed
- ¼ cup green olives, pitted and sliced
- A handful parsley, chopped

Directions:

1. Heat up a pan with the oil over medium-high heat, add the chicken, garlic, salt and pepper and brown for 2 minutes on each side.
2. Add the rest of the ingredients, toss, bring the mix to a simmer and cook over medium heat for 13 minutes.
3. Divide the mix between plates and serve.

Nutrition: calories 135, fat 5.8, fiber 3.4, carbs 12.1, protein 9.6

Chicken Bake

Preparation time: 10 minutes
Cooking time: 30 minutes
Servings: 4
Ingredients:

- 1 and ½ pounds chicken thighs, skinless, boneless and cubed
- 2 garlic cloves, minced
- 1 tablespoon oregano, chopped
- 2 tablespoons olive oil
- 1 tablespoon red wine vinegar
- ½ cup canned artichokes, drained and chopped
- 1 red onion, sliced
- 1 pound whole wheat fusili pasta, cooked
- ½ cup canned white beans, drained and rinsed
- ½ cup parsley, chopped
- 1 cup mozzarella, shredded
- Salt and black pepper to the taste

Directions:

1. Heat up a pan with half of the oil over medium-high heat, add the meat and brown for 5 minutes.
2. Grease a baking pan with the rest of the oil, add the browned chicken, and the rest of the ingredients except the pasta and the mozzarella.
3. Spread the pasta all over and toss gently.
4. Sprinkle the mozzarella on top and bake at 425 degrees F for 25 minutes.
5. Divide the bake between plates and serve.

Nutrition: calories 195, fat 5.8, fiber 3.4, carbs 12.1, protein 11.6

Pesto Chicken Mix

Preparation time: 10 minutes
Cooking time: 40 minutes
Servings: 4
Ingredients:

- 4 chicken breast halves, skinless and boneless
- 3 tomatoes, cubed
- 1 cup mozzarella, shredded
- ½ cup basil pesto
- A pinch of salt and black pepper
- Cooking spray

Directions:

1. Grease a baking dish lined with parchment paper with the cooking spray.
2. In a bowl, mix the chicken with salt, pepper and the pesto and rub well.
3. Place the chicken on the baking sheet, top with tomatoes and shredded mozzarella and bake at 400 degrees F for 40 minutes.
4. Divide the mix between plates and serve with a side salad.

Nutrition: calories 341, fat 20, fiber 1, carbs 4, protein 32

Chicken Wrap

Preparation time: 10 minutes
Cooking time: 0 minutes
Servings: 2
Ingredients:

- 2 whole wheat tortilla flatbreads
- 6 chicken breast slices, skinless, boneless, cooked and shredded
- A handful baby spinach
- 2 provolone cheese slices
- 4 tomato slices
- 10 kalamata olives, pitted and sliced
- 1 red onion, sliced
- 2 tablespoons roasted peppers, chopped

Directions:

1. Arrange the tortillas on a working surface, and divide the chicken and the other ingredients on each.
2. Roll the tortillas and serve them right away.

Nutrition: calories 190, fat 6.8, fiber 3.5, carbs 15.1, protein 6.6

Chicken and Artichokes

Preparation time: 10 minutes
Cooking time: 20 minutes
Servings: 4
Ingredients:

- 2 pounds chicken breast, skinless, boneless and sliced
- A pinch of salt and black pepper
- 4 tablespoons olive oil
- 8 ounces canned roasted artichoke hearts, drained
- 6 ounces sun-dried tomatoes, chopped

- 3 tablespoons capers, drained
- 2 tablespoons lemon juice

Directions:

1. Heat up a pan with half of the oil over medium-high heat, add the artichokes and the other ingredients except the chicken, stir and sauté for 10 minutes.
2. Transfer the mix to a bowl, heat up the pan again with the rest of the oil over medium-high heat, add the meat and cook for 4 minutes on each side.
3. Return the veggie mix to the pan, toss, cook everything for 2-3 minutes more, divide between plates and serve.

Nutrition: calories 552, fat 28, fiber 6, carbs 33, protein 43

Chicken Kebabs

Preparation time: 30 minutes
Cooking time: 20 minutes
Servings: 4
Ingredients:

- 2 chicken breasts, skinless, boneless and cubed
- 1 red bell pepper, cut into squares
- 1 red onion, roughly cut into squares
- 2 teaspoons sweet paprika
- 1 teaspoon nutmeg, ground
- 1 teaspoon Italian seasoning
- ¼ teaspoon smoked paprika
- A pinch of salt and black pepper
- ¼ teaspoon cardamom, ground
- Juice of 1 lemon
- 3 garlic cloves, minced
- ½ cup olive oil

Directions:

1. In a bowl, combine the chicken with the onion, the bell pepper and the other ingredients, toss well, cover the bowl and keep in the fridge for 30 minutes.
2. Assemble skewers with chicken, peppers and the onions, place them on your preheated grill and cook over medium heat for 8 minutes on each side.
3. Divide the kebabs between plates and serve with a side salad.

Nutrition: calories 262, fat 14, fiber 2, carbs 14, protein 20

Chicken Salad and Mustard Dressing

Preparation time: 10 minutes
Cooking time: 0 minutes
Servings: 8
Ingredients:

- 1 cup rotisserie chicken, skinless, boneless and cubed
- ½ cup sun-dried tomatoes, chopped
- ½ cup marinated artichoke hearts, drained and chopped
- 1 cucumber, chopped
- 1/3 cup kalamata olives, pitted and sliced
- 2 cups baby arugula
- ¼ cup parsley, chopped
- 1 avocado, peeled, pitted and cubed

- ½ cup feta cheese, crumbled
- 4 tablespoons red wine vinegar
- 2 tablespoons Dijon mustard
- 1 teaspoon basil, dried
- 1 garlic clove, minced
- 2 teaspoons honey
- ½ cup olive oil
- Salt and black pepper to the taste
- 3 tablespoons lemon juice

Directions:

1. In a salad bowl, mix the chicken with the tomatoes, artichokes, cucumber, olives, arugula, parsley and the avocado and toss.
2. In a different bowl, mix the vinegar with the mustard and the remaining ingredients except the cheese, whisk well, add to the salad, and toss.
3. Sprinkle the cheese on top and serve.

Nutrition: calories 326, fat 21.7, fiber 1.7, carbs 24.9, protein 8.8

Chili Chicken Mix

Preparation time: 10 minutes
Cooking time: 18 minutes
Servings: 4
Ingredients:

- 2 pounds chicken thighs, skinless and boneless
- 2 tablespoons olive oil
- 2 cups yellow onion, chopped
- 1 teaspoon onion powder
- 1 teaspoon smoked paprika
- 1 teaspoon chili pepper
- ½ teaspoon coriander seeds, ground
- 2 teaspoons oregano, dried
- 2 teaspoon parsley flakes
- 30 ounces canned tomatoes, chopped
- ½ cup black olives, pitted and halved

Directions:

1. Set the instant pot on Sauté mode, add the oil, heat it up, add the onion, onion powder and the rest of the ingredients except the tomatoes, olives and the chicken, stir and sauté for 10 minutes.
2. Add the chicken, tomatoes and the olives, put the lid on and cook on High for 8 minutes.
3. Release the pressure naturally 10 minutes, divide the mix into bowls and serve.

Nutrition: calories 153, fat 8, fiber 2, carbs 9, protein 12

Chicken Pilaf

Preparation time: 10 minutes
Cooking time: 30 minutes
Servings: 4
Ingredients:

- 4 tablespoons avocado oil
- 2 pounds chicken breasts, skinless, boneless and cubed
- ½ cup yellow onion, chopped
- 4 garlic cloves, minced
- 8 ounces brown rice
- 4 cups chicken stock

- ½ cup kalamata olives, pitted
- ½ cup tomatoes, cubed
- 6 ounces baby spinach
- ½ cup feta cheese, crumbled
- A pinch of salt and black pepper
- 1 tablespoon marjoram, chopped
- 1 tablespoon basil, chopped
- Juice of ½ lemon
- ¼ cup pine nuts, toasted

Directions:
1. Heat up a pot with 1 tablespoon avocado oil over medium-high heat, add the chicken, some salt and pepper, brown for 5 minutes on each side and transfer to a bowl.
2. Heat up the pot again with the rest of the avocado oil over medium heat, add the onion and garlic and sauté for 3 minutes.
3. Add the rice, the rest of the ingredients except the pine nuts, also return the chicken, toss, bring to a simmer and cook over medium heat for 20 minutes.
4. Divide the mix between plates, top each serving with some pine nuts and serve.

Nutrition: calories 283, fat 12.5, fiber 8.2, carbs 21.5, protein 13.4

Chicken and Sweet Potatoes

Preparation time: 10 minutes
Cooking time: 40 minutes
Servings: 6
Ingredients:
- 2 pounds chicken breasts, skinless, boneless and sliced
- 2 tablespoons harissa seasoning
- Juice of 1 lemon
- Zest of 1 lemon, grated
- ¼ cup olive oil
- Salt and black pepper to the taste
- 2 sweet potatoes, peeled and roughly cubed
- 1 sweet onion, chopped
- ½ cup feta cheese, crumbled
- ½ cup green olives, pitted and smashed

Directions:
1. In a roasting pan, combine the chicken with the seasoning and the rest of the ingredients except the cheese and the olives, toss and bake at 425 degrees F for 40 minutes.
2. In a bowl, combine the cheese with the smashed olives and stir well.
3. Divide the chicken and sweet potatoes between plates, top each serving with the cheese and olives mix and serve right away.

Nutrition: calories 303, fat 9.5, fiber 9.2, carbs 21.5, protein 13.6

Paprika Chicken and Pineapple Mix

Preparation time: 10 minutes
Cooking time: 15 minutes
Servings: 4
Ingredients:
- 2 cups pineapple, peeled and cubed

- 2 tablespoons olive oil
- 1 tablespoon smoked paprika
- 2 pounds chicken breasts, skinless, boneless and cubed
- A pinch of salt and black pepper
- 1 tablespoon chives, chopped

Directions:
1. Heat up a pan with the oil over medium-high heat, add the chicken, salt and pepper and brown for 4 minutes on each side.
2. Add the rest of the ingredients, toss, cook for 7 minutes more, divide everything between plates and serve with a side salad.

Nutrition: calories 264, fat 13.2, fiber 8.3, carbs 25.1, protein 15.4

Chicken and Cashews Mix

Preparation time: 10 minutes
Cooking time: 30 minutes
Servings: 4
Ingredients:
- 1 and ½ pounds chicken breasts, skinless, boneless and roughly cubed
- 4 spring onions, chopped
- 2 tablespoons olive oil
- 2 carrots, peeled and sliced
- ¼ cup mayonnaise
- ½ cup Greek yogurt
- 1 cup cashews, toasted and chopped
- A pinch of salt and black pepper

Directions:
1. Heat up a pan with the oil over medium-high heat, add the chicken and cook for 4 minutes on each side.
2. Add the onions, carrots and the rest of the ingredients except the cashews, toss, bring to a simmer and cook over medium heat for 20 minutes.
3. Divide the mix into bowls and serve with the cashews sprinkled in top.

Nutrition: calories 304, fat 13.2, fiber 6.5, carbs 19.1, protein 15.4

Chicken, Corn and Peppers

Preparation time: 5 minutes
Cooking time: 1 hour
Servings: 4
Ingredients:
- 2 pounds chicken breast, skinless, boneless and cubed
- 2 tablespoons olive oil
- 2 garlic cloves, minced
- 1 red onion, chopped
- 2 red bell peppers, chopped
- ¼ teaspoon cumin, ground
- 2 cups corn
- ½ cup chicken stock
- 1 teaspoon chili powder
- ¼ cup cilantro, chopped

Directions:

1. Heat up a pot with the oil over medium-high heat, add the chicken and brown for 4 minutes on each side.
2. Add the onion and the garlic and sauté for 5 minutes more.
3. Add the rest of the ingredients, stir, bring to a simmer over medium heat and cook for 45 minutes.
4. Divide into bowls and serve.
Nutrition: calories 332, fat 16.1, fiber 8.4, carbs 25.4, protein 17.4

Chicken and Apples Mix

Preparation time: 10 minutes
Cooking time: 40 minutes
Servings: 4
Ingredients:
- ½ cup chicken stock
- 1 red onion, sliced
- ½ cup tomato sauce
- 2 green apples, cored and chopped
- 1 pound breast, skinless, boneless and cubed
- 1 teaspoon thyme, chopped
- 1 and ½ tablespoons olive oil
- 1 tablespoon chives, chopped

Directions:
1. In a roasting pan, combine the chicken with the tomato sauce, apples and the rest of the ingredients except the chives, introduce the pan in the oven and bake at 425 degrees F for 40 minutes.
2. Divide the mix between plates, sprinkle the chives on top and serve.
Nutrition: calories 292, fat 16.1, fiber 9.4, carbs 15.4, protein 16.4

Walnut Turkey and Peaches

Preparation time: 10 minutes
Cooking time: 1 hour
Servings: 4
Ingredients:
- 2 turkey breasts, skinless, boneless and sliced
- ¼ cup chicken stock
- 1 tablespoon walnuts, chopped
- 1 red onion, chopped
- Salt and black pepper to the taste
- 2 tablespoons olive oil
- 4 peaches, pitted and cut into quarters
- 1 tablespoon cilantro, chopped

Directions:
1. In a roasting pan greased with the oil, combine the turkey and the onion and the rest of the ingredients except the cilantro, introduce in the oven and bake at 390 degrees F for 1 hours.
2. Divide the mix between plates, sprinkle the cilantro on top and serve.
Nutrition: calories 500, fat 14, fiber 3, carbs 15, protein 10

Balsamic Turkey Bites and Apricots

Preparation time: 5 minutes
Cooking time: 1 hour
Servings: 4

Ingredients:
- 1 cup apricots, pitted and cubed
- ¼ cup chicken stock
- 1 big turkey breast, skinless, boneless and cubed
- 1 tablespoon balsamic vinegar
- 1 sweet onion, chopped
- ¼ teaspoon red pepper flakes
- 2 tablespoons olive oil
- Salt and black pepper to the taste
- 2 tablespoons parsley, chopped

Directions:
1. Heat up a pan with the oil over medium-high heat, add the turkey and brown for 3 minutes on each side.
2. Add the onion, pepper flakes and the vinegar and cook for 5 minutes more.
3. Add the remaining ingredients except the parsley, toss, introduce the pan in the oven and bake at 380 degrees F for 50 minutes.
4. Divide the mix between plates and serve with the parsley sprinkled on top.
Nutrition: calories 292, fat 16.7, fiber 8.6, carbs 24.8, protein 14.4

Chipotle Turkey and Tomatoes

Preparation time: 10 minutes
Cooking time: 1 hour
Servings: 4
Ingredients:
- 2 pounds cherry tomatoes, halved
- 3 tablespoons olive oil
- 1 red onion, roughly chopped
- 1 big turkey breast, skinless, boneless and sliced
- 3 garlic cloves, chopped
- 3 red chili peppers, chopped
- 4 tablespoons chipotle paste
- Zest of ½ lemon, grated
- Juice of 1 lemon
- Salt and black pepper to the taste
- A handful coriander, chopped

Directions:
3. Heat up a pan with the oil over medium-high heat, add the turkey slices, cook for 4 minutes on each side and transfer to a roasting pan.
4. Heat up the pan again over medium-high heat, add the onion, garlic and chili peppers and sauté for 2 minutes.
5. Add chipotle paste, sauté for 3 minutes more and pour over the turkey slices.
6. Toss the turkey slices with the chipotle mix, also add the rest of the ingredients except the coriander, introduce in the oven and bake at 400 degrees F for 45 minutes.
7. Divide everything between plates, sprinkle the coriander on top and serve.
Nutrition: calories 264, fat 13.2, fiber 8.7, carbs 23.9, protein 33.2

Parmesan Chicken and Cream

Preparation time: 10 minutes
Cooking time: 25 minutes
Servings: 4
Ingredients:
- 1 and ½ pounds chicken breasts, skinless, boneless and cubed
- 1 tablespoon olive oil
- 1 teaspoon coriander, ground
- 1 teaspoon parsley flakes
- 2 garlic cloves, minced
- 1 cup heavy cream
- Salt and black pepper to the taste
- ¼ cup parmesan cheese, grated
- 1 tablespoon basil, chopped

Directions:
1. Heat up a pan with the oil over medium high-heat, add the chicken, salt and pepper and cook for 3 minutes on each side.
2. Add the garlic and cook for 1 more minute.
3. Add the rest of the ingredients except the parmesan and basil, cook everything over medium heat for 20 minutes, and divide between plates.
4. Sprinkle the basil and the parmesan on top and serve.

Nutrition: calories 249, fat 16.6, fiber 7.5, carbs 24.5, protein 25.3

Oregano Chicken and Zucchini Pan

Preparation time: 10 minutes
Cooking time: 30 minutes
Servings: 4
Ingredients:
- 2 cups tomatoes, peeled and crushed
- 1 and ½ pounds chicken breast, boneless, skinless and cubed
- 2 tablespoons olive oil
- Salt and black pepper to the taste
- 1 small yellow onion, sliced
- 2 garlic cloves, minced
- 2 zucchinis, sliced
- 2 tablespoons oregano, chopped
- 1 cup chicken stock

Directions:
1. Heat up a pan with the oil over medium-high heat, add the chicken and brown for 3 minute son each side.
2. Add the onion and the garlic and sauté for 4 minutes more.
3. Add the rest of the ingredients except the oregano, bring to a simmer and cook over medium heat and cook for 20 minutes.
4. Divide the mix between plates, sprinkle the oregano on top and serve.

Nutrition: calories 228, fat 9.5, fiber 9.1, carbs 15.6, protein 18.6

Creamy Chicken and Grapes

Preparation time: 10 minutes
Cooking time: 20 minutes

Servings: 4
Ingredients:
- 1 and ½ pounds chicken breasts, skinless, boneless and cubed
- ½ cup almonds, chopped
- 1 cup green grapes, seedless and halved
- 2 tablespoons olive oil
- Salt and black pepper to the taste
- 1 cup heavy cream
- 1 tablespoon chives, chopped

Directions:
1. Heat up a pan with the oil over medium-high heat, add the chicken and brown for 3 minutes on each side.
2. Add the grapes and the rest of the ingredients, bring to a simmer and cook over medium heat fro 15 minutes more.
3. Divide everything into bowls and serve.

Nutrition: calories

Chicken and Ginger Cucumbers Mix

Preparation time: 10 minutes
Cooking time: 20 minutes
Servings: 4
Ingredients:
- 4 chicken breasts, boneless, skinless and cubed
- 2 cucumbers, cubed
- Salt and black pepper to the taste
- 1 tablespoon ginger, grated
- 1 tablespoon garlic, minced
- 2 tablespoons balsamic vinegar
- 3 tablespoons olive oil
- ¼ teaspoon chili paste
- ½ cup chicken stock
- ½ tablespoon lime juice
- 1 tablespoon chives, chopped

Directions:
1. Heat up a pan with the oil over medium-high heat, add the chicken and brown for 3 minutes on each side.
2. Add the cucumbers, salt, pepper and the rest of the ingredients except the chives, bring to a simmer and cook over medium heat for 15 minutes.
3. Divide the mix between plates and serve with the chives sprinkled on top.

Nutrition: calories 288, fat 9.5, fiber 12.1, carbs 25.6, protein 28.6

Turmeric Chicken and Eggplant Mix

Preparation time: 10 minutes
Cooking time: 30 minutes
Servings: 4
Ingredients:
- 2 cups eggplant, cubed
- Salt and black pepper to the taste
- 2 tablespoons olive oil
- 1 cup yellow onion, chopped
- 2 tablespoons garlic, minced
- 2 tablespoons hot paprika
- 1 teaspoon turmeric powder

- 1 and ½ tablespoons oregano, chopped
- 1 cup chicken stock
- 1 pound chicken breast, skinless, boneless and cubed
- 1 cup half and half
- 1 tablespoon lemon juice

Directions:
1. Heat up a pan with the oil over medium-high heat, add the chicken and brown for 4 minutes on each side.
2. Add the eggplant, onion and garlic and sauté for 5 minutes more.
3. Add the rest of the ingredients, bring to a simmer and cook over medium heat for 16 minutes.
4. Divide the mix between plates and serve.

Nutrition: calories 392, fat 11.6, fiber 8.3, carbs 21.1, protein 24.2

Tomato Chicken and Lentils

Preparation time: 10 minutes
Cooking time: 1 hour
Servings: 8
Ingredients:
- 2 tablespoons olive oil
- 2 celery stalks, chopped
- 1 red onion, chopped
- 2 tablespoons tomato paste
- 2 garlic cloves, chopped
- ½ cup chicken stock
- 2 cups French lentils
- 1 pound chicken thighs, boneless and skinless
- Salt and black pepper to the taste
- 1 tablespoon cilantro, chopped

Directions:
4. Heat up a Dutch oven with the oil over medium-high heat, add the onion and the garlic and sauté for 2 minutes.
5. Add the chicken and brown for 3 minutes on each side.
6. Add the rest of the ingredients except the cilantro, bring to a simmer and cook over medium-low heat for 45 minutes.
7. Add the cilantro, stir, divide the mix into bowls and serve.

Nutrition: calories 249, fat 9.7, fiber 11.9, carbs 25.3, protein 24.3

Turkey, Leeks and Carrots

Preparation time: 10 minutes
Cooking time: 1 hour
Servings: 4
Ingredients:
- 1 big turkey breast, skinless, boneless and cubed
- 2 tablespoons avocado oil
- Salt and black pepper to the taste
- 1 tablespoon sweet paprika
- ½ cup chicken stock
- 1 leek, sliced
- 1 carrot, sliced
- 1 yellow onion, chopped
- 1 tablespoon lemon juice
- 1 teaspoon cumin, ground
- 1 tablespoon basil, chopped

Directions:
1. Heat up a pan with the oil over medium-high heat, add the turkey and brown for 4 minutes on each side.
2. Add the leeks, carrot and the onion and sauté everything for 5 minutes more.
3. Add the rest of the ingredients, bring to a simmer and cook over medium heat for 40 minutes.
4. Divide the mix between plates and serve.

Nutrition: calories 249, fat 10.7, fiber 11.9, carbs 22.3, protein 17.3

Chicken and Celery Quinoa Mix

Preparation time: 10 minutes
Cooking time: 50 minutes
Servings: 4
Ingredients:
- 4 chicken things, skinless and boneless
- 1 tablespoon olive oil
- Salt and black pepper to the taste
- 2 celery stalks, chopped
- 2 spring onions, chopped
- 2 cups chicken stock
- ½ cup cilantro, chopped
- ½ cup quinoa
- 1 teaspoon lime zest, grated

Directions:
5. Heat up a pot with the oil over medium-high heat, add the chicken and brown for 4 minutes on each side.
6. Add the onion and the celery, stir and sauté everything for 5 minutes more.
7. Add the rest of the ingredients, toss, bring to a simmer and cook over medium-low heat for 35 minutes.
8. Divide everything between plates and serve.

Nutrition: calories 241, fat 12.6, fiber 9.5, carbs 15.6, protein 34.1

Herbed Chicken

Preparation time: 10 minutes
Cooking time: 40 minutes
Servings: 4
Ingredients:
- 2 chicken breasts, skinless, boneless and sliced
- 2 red onions, chopped
- 2 tablespoons olive oil
- 2 garlic cloves, minced
- ½ cup chicken stock
- 1 teaspoon oregano, dried
- 1 teaspoon basil, dried
- 1 teaspoon rosemary, dried
- 1 cup canned tomatoes, chopped
- Salt and black pepper to the taste

Directions:

1.   Heat up a pot with the oil over medium-high heat, add the chicken and brown for 4 minutes on each side.
2.   Add the garlic and the onions and sauté for 5 minutes more.
3.   Add the rest of the ingredients, bring to a simmer and cook over medium heat for 25 minutes.
4.   Divide everything between plates and serve.
Nutrition: calories 251, fat 11.6, fiber 15.5, carbs 15.6, protein 9.1

Chives Chicken and Radishes
Preparation time: 10 minutes
Cooking time: 30 minutes
Servings: 4
Ingredients:
- 2 chicken breasts, skinless, boneless and cubed
- Salt and black pepper to the taste
- 1 tablespoon olive oil
- 1 cup chicken stock
- ½ cup tomato sauce
- ½ pound red radishes, cubed
- 2 tablespoon chives, chopped

Directions:
1.   Heat up a Dutch oven with the oil over medium-high heat, add the chicken and brown for 4 minutes on each side.
2.   Add the rest of the ingredients except the chives, bring to a simmer and cook over medium heat for 20 minutes.
3.   Divide the mix between plates, sprinkle the chives on top and serve.
Nutrition: calories 277, fat 15, fiber 9.3, carbs 20.9, protein 33.2

Feta Chicken and Cabbage
Preparation time: 10 minutes
Cooking time: 25 minutes
Servings: 4
Ingredients:
- 2 chicken breasts, skinless, boneless and cut into strips
- 1 red cabbage, shredded
- 2 tablespoons olive oil
- Salt and black pepper to the taste
- 2 tablespoons balsamic vinegar
- 1 and ½ cups tomatoes, cubed
- 1 tablespoon chives, chopped
- ¼ cup feta cheese, crumbled

Directions:
1.   Heat up a pan with the oil over medium-high heat, add the chicken and brown for 5 minutes.
2.   Add the rest of the ingredients except the cheese, and cook over medium heat for 20 minutes stirring often.
3.   Add the cheese, toss, divide everything between plates and serve.
Nutrition: calories 277, fat 15, fiber 8.6, carbs 14.9, protein 14.2

Garlic Chicken and Endives
Preparation time: 10 minutes
Cooking time: 15 minutes
Servings: 4
Ingredients:
- 1 pound chicken breasts, skinless, boneless and cubed
- 2 endives, sliced
- 2 tablespoons olive oil
- 4 garlic cloves, minced
- ½ cup chicken stock
- 2 tablespoons parmesan, grated
- 1 tablespoon parsley, chopped
- Salt and black pepper to the taste

Directions:
1.   Heat up a pan with the oil over medium-high heat, add the chicken and cook for 5 minutes.
2.   Add the endives, garlic, the stock, salt and pepper, stir, bring to a simmer and cook over medium-high heat for 10 minutes.
3.   Add the parmesan and the parsley, toss gently, divide everything between plates and serve.
Nutrition: calories 280, fat 9.2, fiber 10.8, carbs 21.6, protein 33.8

Brown Rice, Chicken and Scallions
Preparation time: 10 minutes
Cooking time: 30 minutes
Servings: 4
Ingredients:
- 1 and ½ cups brown rice
- 3 cups chicken stock
- 2 tablespoon balsamic vinegar
- 1 pound chicken breast, boneless, skinless and cubed
- 6 scallions, chopped
- Salt and black pepper to the taste
- 1 tablespoon sweet paprika
- 2 tablespoons avocado oil

Directions:
1.   Heat up a pan with the oil over medium-high heat, add the chicken and brown for 5 minutes.
2.   Add the scallions and sauté for 5 minutes more.
3.   Add the rice and the rest of the ingredients, bring to a simmer and cook over medium heat for 20 minutes.
4.   Stir the mix, divide everything between plates and serve.
Nutrition: calories 300, fat 9.2, fiber 11.8, carbs 18.6, protein 23.8

Creamy Chicken And Mushrooms
Preparation time: 10 minutes
Cooking time: 30 minutes
Servings: 4
Ingredients:
- 1 red onion, chopped
- 1 tablespoon olive oil
- 2 garlic cloves, minced
- 2 carrots chopped

- Salt and black pepper to the taste
- 1 tablespoon thyme, chopped
- 1 and ½ cups chicken stock
- ½ pound Bella mushrooms, sliced
- 1 cup heavy cream
- 2 chicken breasts, skinless, boneless and cubed
- 2 tablespoons chives, chopped
- 1 tablespoon parsley, chopped

Directions:
1. Heat up a Dutch oven with the oil over medium-high heat, add the onion and the garlic and sauté for 5 minutes.
2. Add the chicken and the mushrooms, and sauté for 10 minutes more.
3. Add the rest of the ingredients except the chives and the parsley, bring to a simmer and cook over medium heat for 15 minutes.
4. Add the chives and parsley, divide the mix between plates and serve.

Nutrition: calories 275, fat 11.9, fiber 10.6, carbs 26.7, protein 23.7

Curry Chicken, Artichokes and Olives

Preparation time: 5 minutes
Cooking time: 7 hours
Servings: 6
Ingredients:
- 2 pounds chicken breasts, boneless, skinless and cubed
- 12 ounces canned artichoke hearts, drained
- 1 cup chicken stock
- 1 red onion, chopped
- 1 tablespoon white wine vinegar
- 1 cup kalamata olives, pitted and chopped
- 1 tablespoon curry powder
- 2 teaspoons basil, dried
- Salt and black pepper to the taste
- ¼ cup rosemary, chopped

Directions:
1. In your slow cooker, combine the chicken with the artichokes, olives and the rest of the ingredients, put the lid on and cook on Low for 7 hours.
2. Divide the mix between plates and serve hot.

Nutrition: calories 275, fat 11.9, fiber 7.6, carbs 19.7, protein 18.7

Slow Cooked Chicken and Capers Mix

Preparation time: 5 minutes
Cooking time: 7 hours
Servings: 4
Ingredients:
- 2 chicken breasts, skinless, boneless and halved
- 2 cups canned tomatoes, crushed
- 2 garlic cloves, minced
- 1 yellow onion, chopped
- 2 cups chicken stock
- 2 tablespoons capers, drained
- ¼ cup rosemary, chopped
- Salt and black pepper to the taste

Directions:
1. In your slow cooker, combine the chicken with the tomatoes, capers and the rest of the ingredients, put the lid on and cook on Low for 7 hours.
2. Divide the mix between plates and serve.

Nutrition: calories 292, fat 9.4, fiber 11.8, carbs 25.1, protein 36.4

Turkey and Chickpeas

Preparation time: 5 minutes
Cooking time: 5 hours
Servings: 4
Ingredients:
- 2 tablespoons avocado oil
- 1 big turkey breast, skinless, boneless and roughly cubed
- Salt and black pepper to the taste
- 1 red onion, chopped
- 15 ounces canned chickpeas, drained and rinsed
- 15 ounces canned tomatoes, chopped
- 1 cup kalamata olives, pitted and halved
- 2 tablespoons lime juice
- 1 teaspoon oregano, dried

Directions:
1. Heat up a pan with the oil over medium-high heat, add the meat and the onion, brown for 5 minutes and transfer to a slow cooker.
2. Add the rest of the ingredients, put the lid on and cook on High for 5 hours.
3. Divide between plates and serve right away!

Nutrition: calories 352, fat 14.4, fiber 11.8, carbs 25.1, protein 26.4

Chicken Wings and Dates Mix

Preparation time: 10 minutes
Cooking time: 1 hour
Servings: 6
Ingredients:
- 12 chicken wings, halved
- 2 garlic cloves, minced
- Juice of 1 lime
- Zest of 1 lime
- 2 tablespoons avocado oil
- 1 cup dates, pitted and halved
- 1 teaspoon cumin, ground
- Salt and black pepper to the taste
- ½ cup chicken stock
- 1 tablespoon chives, chopped

Directions:
1. In a roasting pan, combine the chicken wings with the garlic, lime juice and the rest of the ingredients, toss, introduce in the oven and bake at 360 degrees F for 1 hour.
2. Divide everything between plates and serve with a side salad.

Nutrition: calories 294, fat 19.4, fiber 11.8, carbs 21.4, protein 17.5

Creamy Coriander Chicken

Preparation time: 10 minutes
Cooking time: 55 minutes
Servings: 4
Ingredients:
- 2 chicken breasts, boneless, skinless and halved
- 2 tablespoons avocado oil
- ½ teaspoon hot paprika
- 1 cup chicken stock
- 1 tablespoon almonds, chopped
- 2 spring onions, chopped
- 2 garlic cloves, minced
- ¼ cup heavy cream
- A handful coriander, chopped
- Salt and black pepper to the taste

Directions:
1. Grease a roasting pan with the oil, add the chicken, paprika and the rest of the ingredients except the coriander and the heavy cream, toss, introduce in the oven and bake at 360 degrees F for 40 minutes.
2. Add the cream and the coriander, toss, bake for 15 minutes more, divide between plates and serve.
Nutrition: calories 225, fat 8.9, fiber 10.2, carbs 20.8, protein 17.5

Lime Turkey and Avocado Mix

Preparation time: 10 minutes
Cooking time: 1 hour and 10 minutes
Servings: 2
Ingredients:
- 2 tablespoons olive oil
- 1 turkey breast, boneless, skinless and halved
- 2 ounces cherry tomatoes, halved
- A handful coriander, chopped
- Juice of 1 lime
- Zest of 1 lime, grated
- Salt and black pepper to the taste
- 2 spring onions, chopped
- 2 avocadoes, pitted, peeled and cubed

Directions:
1. In a roasting pan, combine the turkey with the oil and the rest of the ingredients, introduce in the oven and bake at 370 degrees F for 1 hour and 10 minutes.
2. Divide between plates and serve.
Nutrition: calories 301, fat 8.9, fiber 10.2, carbs 19.8, protein 13.5

Peanut and Chives Chicken Mix

Preparation time: 10 minutes
Cooking time: 25 minutes
Servings: 4
Ingredients:
- 4 chicken breast halves, skinless and boneless
- Salt and black pepper to the taste
- 2 tablespoons olive oil
- 2 tablespoons peanuts, chopped
- 1 tablespoon chives, chopped
- ½ cup tomato sauce

- ½ cup chicken stock

Directions:
1. Heat up a pan with the oil over medium-high heat, add the chicken and brown for 4 minutes on each side.
2. Add the rest of the ingredients, bring to a simmer and cook over medium heat for 16 minutes.
3. Divide the mix between plates and serve.
Nutrition: calories 294, fat 12.1, fiber 9.2, carbs 25.6, protein 35.4

Turkey and Salsa Verde

Preparation time: 10 minutes
Cooking time: 50 minutes
Servings: 4
Ingredients:
- 1 big turkey breast, skinless, boneless and cubed
- 1 and ½ cups Salsa Verde
- Salt and black pepper to the taste
- 1 tablespoon olive oil
- 1 and ½ cups feta cheese, crumbled
- ¼ cup cilantro, chopped

Directions:
1. In a roasting pan greased with the oil combine the turkey with the salsa, salt and pepper and bake 400 degrees F for 50 minutes.
2. Add the cheese and the cilantro, toss gently, divide everything between plates and serve.
Nutrition: calories 332, fat 15.4, fiber 10.5, carbs 22.1, protein 34.5

Basil Turkey and Zucchinis

Preparation time: 10 minutes
Cooking time: 1 hour
Servings: 4
Ingredients:
- 2 tablespoons avocado oil
- 1 pound turkey breast, skinless, boneless and sliced
- Salt and black pepper to the taste
- 3 garlic cloves, minced
- 2 zucchinis, sliced
- 1 cup chicken stock
- ¼ cup heavy cream
- 2 tablespoons basil, chopped

Directions:
1. Heat up a pot with the oil over medium-high heat, add the turkey and brown for 5 minutes on each side.
2. Add the garlic and cook everything for 1 minute.
3. Add the rest of the ingredients except the basil, toss gently, bring to a simmer and cook over medium-low heat for 50 minutes.
4. Add the basil, toss, divide the mix between plates and serve.
Nutrition: calories 262, fat 9.8, fiber 12.2, carbs 25.8, protein 14.6

Duck and Tomato Sauce

Preparation time: 10 minutes

Cooking time: 2 hours
Servings: 4
Ingredients:
- 4 duck legs
- 2 yellow onions, sliced
- 4 garlic cloves, minced
- ¼ cup parsley, chopped
- A pinch of salt and black pepper
- 1 teaspoon herbs de Provence
- 1 cup tomato sauce
- 2 cups black olives, pitted and sliced

Directions:
1. In a baking dish, combine the duck legs with the onions, garlic and the rest of the ingredients, introduce in the oven and bake at 370 degrees F for 2 hours.
2. Divide the mix between plates and serve.
Nutrition: calories 300, fat 13.5, fiber 9.2, carbs 16.7, protein 15.2

Cinnamon Duck Mix

Preparation time: 10 minutes
Cooking time: 20 minutes
Servings: 4
Ingredients:
- 4 duck breasts, boneless and skin scored
- Salt and black pepper to the taste
- 1 teaspoon cinnamon powder
- ½ cup chicken stock
- 3 tablespoons chives, chopped
- 2 tablespoons parsley, chopped
- 1 tablespoon olive oil
- 3 tablespoons balsamic vinegar
- 2 red onions, chopped

Directions:
1. Heat up a pan with the oil over medium-high heat, add the duck skin side down and cook for 5 minutes.
2. Add the cinnamon and the rest of the ingredients except the chives and cook for 5 minutes more.
3. Flip the duck breasts again, bring the whole mix to a simmer and cook over medium heat for 10 minutes.
4. Add the chives, divide everything between plates and serve.
Nutrition: calories 310, fat 13.5, fiber 9.2, carbs 16.7, protein 15.2

Duck and Orange Warm Salad

Preparation time: 10 minutes
Cooking time: 25 minutes
Servings: 4
Ingredients:
- 2 tablespoons balsamic vinegar
- 2 oranges, peeled and cut into segments
- 1 teaspoon orange zest, grated
- 1 tablespoons orange juice
- 3 shallot, minced
- 2 tablespoons olive oil

- Salt and black pepper to the taste
- 2 duck breasts, boneless and skin scored
- 2 cups baby arugula
- 2 tablespoons chives, chopped

Directions:
1. Heat up a pan with the oil over medium-high heat, add the duck breasts skin side down and brown for 5 minutes.
2. Flip the duck, add the shallot, and the other ingredients except the arugula, orange and the chives, and cook for 15 minutes more.
3. Transfer the duck breasts to a cutting board, cool down, cut into strips and put in a salad bowl.
4. Add the remaining ingredients, toss and serve warm.
Nutrition: calories 304, fat 15.4, fiber 12.6, carbs 25.1, protein 36.4

Orange Duck and Celery

Preparation time: 10 minutes
Cooking time: 40 minutes
Servings: 4
Ingredients:
- 2 duck legs, boneless, skinless
- 1 tablespoon avocado oil
- 1 cup chicken stock
- Salt and black pepper to the taste
- 4 celery ribs, roughly chopped
- 2 garlic cloves, minced
- 1 red onion, chopped
- 2 teaspoons thyme, dried
- 2 tablespoons tomato paste
- Zest of 1 orange, grated
- Juice of 2 oranges
- 3 oranges, peeled and cut into segments

Directions:
1. Grease a roasting pan with the oil, add the duck legs, the stock, salt, pepper and the other ingredients, toss a bit and bake at 450 degrees F for 40 minutes.
2. Divide everything between plates and serve warm.
Nutrition: calories 294, fat 12.4, fiber 11.3, carbs 25.5, protein 16.4

Duck and Blackberries

Preparation time: 10 minutes
Cooking time: 25 minutes
Servings: 4
Ingredients:
- 4 duck breasts, boneless and skin scored
- 2 tablespoons balsamic vinegar
- Salt and black pepper to the taste
- 1 cup chicken stock
- 4 ounces blackberries
- ¼ cup chicken stock
- 2 tablespoons avocado oil

Directions:
1. Heat up a pan with the avocado oil over medium-high heat, add duck breasts, skin side down and cook for 5 minutes.

2. Flip the duck, add the rest of the ingredients, bring to a simmer and cook over medium heat for 20 minutes.
3. Divide everything between plates and serve.
Nutrition: calories 239, fat 10.5, fiber 10.2, carbs 21.1, protein 33.3

Ginger Duck Mix

Preparation time: 10 minutes
Cooking time: 1 hour and 50 minutes
Servings: 4
Ingredients:
- 4 duck legs, boneless
- 4 shallots, chopped
- 2 tablespoons olive oil
- 1 tablespoon ginger, grated
- 2 tablespoons rosemary, chopped
- 1 cup chicken stock
- 1 tablespoon chives, chopped

Directions:
1. In a roasting pan, combine the duck legs with the shallots and the rest of the ingredients except the chives, toss, introduce in the oven at 250 degrees F and bake for 1 hour and 30 minutes.
2. Divide the mix between plates, sprinkle the chives on top and serve.
Nutrition: calories 299, fat 10.2, fiber 9.2, carbs 18.1, protein 17.3

Duck, Cucumber and Mango Salad

Preparation time: 10 minutes
Cooking time: 50 minutes
Servings: 4
Ingredients:
- Zest of 1 orange, grated
- 2 big duck breasts, boneless and skin scored
- 2 tablespoons olive oil
- Salt and black pepper to the taste
- 1 tablespoon fish sauce
- 1 tablespoon lime juice
- 1 garlic clove, minced
- 1 Serrano chili, chopped
- 1 small shallot, sliced
- 1 cucumber, sliced
- 2 mangos, peeled and sliced
- ¼ cup oregano, chopped

Directions:
1. Heat up a pan with the oil over medium-high heat, add the duck breasts skin side down and cook for 5 minutes.
2. Add the orange zest, salt, pepper, fish sauce and the rest of the ingredients, bring to a simmer and cook over medium-low heat for 45 minutes.
3. Divide everything between plates and serve.
Nutrition: calories 297, fat 9.1, fiber 10.2, carbs 20.8, protein 16.5

Turkey and Cranberry Sauce

Preparation time: 10 minutes
Cooking time: 50 minutes

Servings: 4
Ingredients:
- 1 cup chicken stock
- 2 tablespoons avocado oil
- ½ cup cranberry sauce
- 1 big turkey breast, skinless, boneless and sliced
- 1 yellow onion, roughly chopped
- Salt and black pepper to the taste

Directions:
1. Heat up a pan with the avocado oil over medium-high heat, add the onion and sauté for 5 minutes.
2. Add the turkey and brown for 5 minutes more.
3. Add the rest of the ingredients, toss, introduce in the oven at 350 degrees F and cook for 40 minutes
Nutrition: calories 382, fat 12.6, fiber 9.6, carbs 26.6, protein 17.6

Sage Turkey Mix

Preparation time: 10 minutes
Cooking time: 40 minutes
Servings: 4
Ingredients:
- 1 big turkey breast, skinless, boneless and roughly cubed
- Juice of 1 lemon
- 2 tablespoons avocado oil
- 1 red onion, chopped
- 2 tablespoons sage, chopped
- 1 garlic clove, minced
- 1 cup chicken stock

Directions:
1. Heat up a pan with the avocado oil over medium-high heat, add the turkey and brown for 3 minutes on each side.
2. Add the rest of the ingredients, bring to a simmer and cook over medium heat for 35 minutes.
3. Divide the mix between plates and serve with a side dish.
Nutrition: calories 382, fat 12.6, fiber 9.6, carbs 16.6, protein 33.2

Turkey and Asparagus Mix

Preparation time: 10 minutes
Cooking time: 30 minutes
Servings: 4
Ingredients:
- 1 bunch asparagus, trimmed and halved
- 1 big turkey breast, skinless, boneless and cut into strips
- 1 teaspoon basil, dried
- 2 tablespoons olive oil
- A pinch of salt and black pepper
- ½ cup tomato sauce
- 1 tablespoon chives, chopped

Directions:
1. Heat up a pan with the oil over medium-high heat, add the turkey and brown for 4 minutes.

2. Add the asparagus and the rest of the ingredients except the chives, bring to a simmer and cook over medium heat for 25 minutes.
3. Add the chives, divide the mix between plates and serve.
Nutrition: calories 337, fat 21.2, fiber 10.2, carbs 21.4, protein 17.6

Herbed Almond Turkey

Preparation time: 10 minutes
Cooking time: 40 minutes
Servings: 4
Ingredients:
- 1 big turkey breast, skinless, boneless and cubed
- 1 tablespoon olive oil
- ½ cup chicken stock
- 1 tablespoon basil, chopped
- 1 tablespoon rosemary, chopped
- 1 tablespoon oregano, chopped
- 1 tablespoon parsley, chopped
- 3 garlic cloves, minced
- ½ cup almonds, toasted and chopped
- 3 cups tomatoes, chopped

Directions:
1. Heat up a pan with the oil over medium-high heat, add the turkey and the garlic and brown for 5 minutes.
2. Add the stock and the rest of the ingredients, bring to a simmer over medium heat and cook for 35 minutes.
3. Divide the mix between plates and serve.
Nutrition: calories 297, fat 11.2, fiber 9.2, carbs 19.4, protein 23.6

Thyme Chicken and Potatoes

Preparation time: 10 minutes
Cooking time: 50 minutes
Servings: 4
Ingredients:
- 1 tablespoon olive oil
- 4 garlic cloves, minced
- A pinch of salt and black pepper
- 2 teaspoons thyme, dried
- 12 small red potatoes, halved
- 2 pounds chicken breast, skinless, boneless and cubed
- 1 cup red onion, sliced
- ¾ cup chicken stock
- 2 tablespoons basil, chopped

Directions:
1. In a baking dish greased with the oil, add the potatoes, chicken and the rest of the ingredients, toss a bit, introduce in the oven and bake at 400 degrees F for 50 minutes.
2. Divide between plates and serve.
Nutrition: calories 281, fat 9.2, fiber 10.9, carbs 21.6, protein 13.6

Turkey, Artichokes and Asparagus

Preparation time: 10 minutes
Cooking time: 30 minutes
Servings: 4
Ingredients:
- 2 turkey breasts, boneless, skinless and halved
- 3 tablespoons olive oil
- 1 and ½ pounds asparagus, trimmed and halved
- 1 cup chicken stock
- A pinch of salt and black pepper
- 1 cup canned artichoke hearts, drained
- ¼ cup kalamata olives, pitted and sliced
- 1 shallot, chopped
- 3 garlic cloves, minced
- 3 tablespoons dill, chopped

Directions:
1. Heat up a pan with the oil over medium-high heat, add the turkey and the garlic and brown for 4 minutes on each side.
2. Add the asparagus, the stock and the rest of the ingredients except the dill, bring to a simmer and cook over medium heat for 20 minutes.
3. Add the dill, divide the mix between plates and serve.
Nutrition: calories 291, fat 16, fiber 10.3, carbs 22.8, protein 34.5

Lemony Turkey and Pine Nuts

Preparation time: 10 minutes
Cooking time: 30 minutes
Servings: 4
Ingredients:
- 2 turkey breasts, boneless, skinless and halved
- A pinch of salt and black pepper
- 2 tablespoons avocado oil
- Juice of 2 lemons
- 1 tablespoon rosemary, chopped
- 3 garlic cloves, minced
- ¼ cup pine nuts, chopped
- 1 cup chicken stock

Directions:
1. Heat up a pan with the oil over medium-high heat, add the garlic and the turkey and brown for 4 minutes on each side.
2. Add the rest of the ingredients, bring to a simmer and cook over medium heat for 20 minutes.
3. Divide the mix between plates and serve with a side salad.
Nutrition: calories 293, fat 12.4, fiber 9.3, carbs 17.8, protein 24.5

Yogurt Chicken and Red Onion Mix

Preparation time: 10 minutes
Cooking time: 30 minutes
Servings: 4
Ingredients:
- 2 pounds chicken breast, skinless, boneless and sliced
- 3 tablespoons olive oil

- ¼ cup Greek yogurt
- 2 garlic cloves, minced
- ½ teaspoon onion powder
- A pinch of salt and black pepper
- 4 red onions, sliced

Directions:
1. In a roasting pan, combine the chicken with the oil, the yogurt and the other ingredients, introduce in the oven at 375 degrees F and bake for 30 minutes.
2. Divide chicken mix between plates and serve hot.
Nutrition: calories 278, fat 15, fiber 9.2, carbs 15.1, protein 23.3

Chicken and Mint Sauce

Preparation time: 10 minutes
Cooking time: 30 minutes
Servings: 4
Ingredients:
- 2 and ½ tablespoons olive oil
- 2 pounds chicken breasts, skinless, boneless and halved
- 3 tablespoons garlic, minced
- 2 tablespoons lemon juice
- 1 tablespoon red wine vinegar
- 1/3 cup Greek yogurt
- 2 tablespoons mint, chopped
- A pinch of salt and black pepper

Directions:
1. In a blender, combine the garlic with the lemon juice and the other ingredients except the oil and the chicken and pulse well.
2. Heat up a pan with the oil over medium-high heat, add the chicken and brown for 3 minutes on each side.
3. Add the mint sauce, introduce in the oven and bake everything at 370 degrees F for 25 minutes.
4. Divide the mix between plates and serve.
Nutrition: calories 278, fat 12, fiber 11.2, carbs 18.1, protein 13.3

Oregano Turkey and Peppers

Preparation time: 10 minutes
Cooking time: 1 hour
Servings: 4
Ingredients:
- 2 red bell peppers, cut into strips
- 2 green bell peppers, cut into strips
- 1 red onion, chopped
- 4 garlic cloves, minced
- ½ cup black olives, pitted and sliced
- 2 cups chicken stock
- 1 big turkey breast, skinless, boneless and cut into strips
- 1 tablespoon oregano, chopped
- ½ cup cilantro, chopped

Directions:
1. In a baking pan, combine the peppers with the turkey and the rest of the ingredients, toss, introduce in the oven at 400 degrees F and roast for 1 hour.

2. Divide everything between plates and serve.
Nutrition: calories 229, fat 8.9, fiber 8.2, carbs 17.8, protein 33.6

Chicken and Mustard Sauce

Preparation time: 10 minutes
Cooking time: 26 minutes
Servings: 4
Ingredients:
- 1/3 cup mustard
- Salt and black pepper to the taste
- 1 red onion, chopped
- 1 tablespoon olive oil
- 1 and ½ cups chicken stock
- 4 chicken breasts, skinless, boneless and halved
- ¼ teaspoon oregano, dried

Directions:
1. Heat up a pan with the stock over medium heat, add the mustard, onion, salt, pepper and the oregano, whisk, bring to a simmer and cook for 8 minutes.
2. Heat up a pan with the oil over medium-high heat, add the chicken and brown for 3 minutes on each side.
3. Add the chicken to the pan with the sauce, toss, simmer everything for 12 minutes more, divide between plates and serve.
Nutrition: calories 247, fat 15.1, fiber 9.1, carbs 16.6, protein 26.1

Chicken and Sausage Mix

Preparation time: 10 minutes
Cooking time: 50 minutes
Servings: 4
Ingredients:
- 2 zucchinis, cubed
- 1 pound Italian sausage, cubed
- 2 tablespoons olive oil
- 1 red bell pepper, chopped
- 1 red onion, sliced
- 2 tablespoons garlic, minced
- 2 chicken breasts, boneless, skinless and halved
- Salt and black pepper to the taste
- ½ cup chicken stock
- 1 tablespoon balsamic vinegar

Directions:
1. Heat up a pan with half of the oil over medium-high heat, add the sausages, brown for 3 minutes on each side and transfer to a bowl.
2. Heat up the pan again with the rest of the oil over medium-high heat, add the chicken and brown for 4 minutes on each side.
3. Return the sausage, add the rest of the ingredients as well, bring to a simmer, introduce in the oven and bake at 400 degrees F for 30 minutes.
4. Divide everything between plates and serve.
Nutrition: calories 293, fat 13.1, fiber 8.1, carbs 16.6, protein 26.1

Coriander and Coconut Chicken

Preparation time: 10 minutes

Cooking time: 30 minutes
Servings: 4
Ingredients:
- 2 pounds chicken thighs, skinless, boneless and cubed
- 2 tablespoons olive oil
- Salt and black pepper to the taste
- 3 tablespoons coconut flesh, shredded
- 1 and ½ teaspoons orange extract
- 1 tablespoon ginger, grated
- ¼ cup orange juice
- 2 tablespoons coriander, chopped
- 1 cup chicken stock
- ¼ teaspoon red pepper flakes

Directions:
1. Heat up a pan with the oil over medium-high heat, add the chicken and brown for 4 minutes on each side.
2. Add salt, pepper and the rest of the ingredients, bring to a simmer and cook over medium heat for 20 minutes.
3. Divide the mix between plates and serve hot.
Nutrition: calories 297, fat 14.4, fiber 9.6, carbs 22, protein 25

Saffron Chicken Thighs and Green Beans

Preparation time: 10 minutes
Cooking time: 25 minutes
Servings: 4
Ingredients:
- 2 pounds chicken thighs, boneless and skinless
- 2 teaspoons saffron powder
- 1 pound green beans, trimmed and halved
- ½ cup Greek yogurt
- Salt and black pepper to the taste
- 1 tablespoon lime juice
- 1 tablespoon dill, chopped

Directions:
1. In a roasting pan, combine the chicken with the saffron, green beans and the rest of the ingredients, toss a bit, introduce in the oven and bake at 400 degrees F for 25 minutes.
2. Divide everything between plates and serve.
Nutrition: calories 274, fat 12.3, fiber 5.3, carbs 20.4, protein 14.3

Chicken and Olives Salsa

Preparation time: 10 minutes
Cooking time: 25 minutes
Servings: 4
Ingredients:
- 2 tablespoon avocado oil
- 4 chicken breast halves, skinless and boneless
- Salt and black pepper to the taste
- 1 tablespoon sweet paprika
- 1 red onion, chopped
- 1 tablespoon balsamic vinegar
- 2 tablespoons parsley, chopped
- 1 avocado, peeled, pitted and cubed

- 2 tablespoons black olives, pitted and chopped

Directions:
1. Heat up your grill over medium-high heat, add the chicken brushed with half of the oil and seasoned with paprika, salt and pepper, cook for 7 minutes on each side and divide between plates.
2. Meanwhile, in a bowl, mix the onion with the rest of the ingredients and the remaining oil, toss, add on top of the chicken and serve.
Nutrition: calories 289, fat 12.4, fiber 9.1, carbs 23.8, protein 14.3

Carrots and Tomatoes Chicken

Preparation time: 10 minutes
Cooking time: 1 hour and 10 minutes
Servings: 4
Ingredients:
- 2 pounds chicken breasts, skinless, boneless and halved
- Salt and black pepper to the taste
- 3 garlic cloves, minced
- 3 tablespoons avocado oil
- 2 shallots, chopped
- 4 carrots, sliced
- 3 tomatoes, chopped
- ¼ cup chicken stock
- 1 tablespoon Italian seasoning
- 1 tablespoon parsley, chopped

Directions:
1. Heat up a pan with the oil over medium-high heat, add the chicken, garlic, salt and pepper and brown for 3 minutes on each side.
2. Add the rest of the ingredients except the parsley, bring to a simmer and cook over medium-low heat for 40 minutes.
3. Add the parsley, divide the mix between plates and serve.
Nutrition: calories 309, fat 12.4, fiber 11.1, carbs 23.8, protein 15.3

Smoked and Hot Turkey Mix

Preparation time: 10 minutes
Cooking time: 40 minutes
Servings: 4
Ingredients:
- 1 red onion, sliced
- 1 big turkey breast, skinless, boneless and roughly cubed
- 1 tablespoon smoked paprika
- 2 chili peppers, chopped
- Salt and black pepper to the taste
- 2 tablespoons olive oil
- ½ cup chicken stock
- 1 tablespoon parsley, chopped
- 1 tablespoon cilantro, chopped

Directions:
1. Grease a roasting pan with the oil, add the turkey, onion, paprika and the rest of the ingredients, toss, introduce in the oven and bake at 425 degrees F for 40 minutes.

2. Divide the mix between plates and serve right away.
Nutrition: calories 310, fat 18.4, fiber 10.4, carbs 22.3, protein 33.4

Spicy Cumin Chicken

Preparation time: 10 minutes
Cooking time: 25 minutes
Servings: 4
Ingredients:
2 teaspoons chili powder
2 and ½ tablespoons olive oil
Salt and black pepper to the taste
1 and ½ teaspoons garlic powder
1 tablespoon smoked paprika
½ cup chicken stock
1 pound chicken breasts, skinless, boneless and halved
2 teaspoons sherry vinegar
2 teaspoons hot sauce
2 teaspoons cumin, ground
½ cup black olives, pitted and sliced
Directions:
1. Heat up a pan with the oil over medium-high heat, add the chicken and brown for 3 minutes on each side.
2. Add the chili powder, salt, pepper, garlic powder and paprika, toss and cook for 4 minutes more.
3. Add the rest of the ingredients, toss, bring to a simmer and cook over medium heat for 15 minutes more.
4. Divide the mix between plates and serve.
Nutrition: calories 230, fat 18.4, fiber 9.4, carbs 15.3, protein 13.4

Chicken with Artichokes and Beans

Preparation time: 10 minutes
Cooking time: 40 minutes
Servings: 4
Ingredients:
- 2 tablespoons olive oil
- 2 chicken breasts, skinless, boneless and halved
- Zest of 1 lemon, grated
- 3 garlic cloves, crushed
- Juice of 1 lemon
- Salt and black pepper to the taste
- 1 tablespoon thyme, chopped
- 6 ounces canned artichokes hearts, drained
- 1 cup canned fava beans, drained and rinsed
- 1 cup chicken stock
- A pinch of cayenne pepper
- Salt and black pepper to the taste
Directions:
1. Heat up a pan with the oil over medium-high heat, add chicken and brown for 5 minutes.
2. Add lemon juice, lemon zest, salt, pepper and the rest of the ingredients, bring to a simmer and cook over medium heat for 35 minutes.
3. Divide the mix between plates and serve right away.

Nutrition: calories 291, fat 14.9, fiber 10.5, carbs 23.8, protein 24.2

Chicken and Olives Tapenade

Preparation time: 10 minutes
Cooking time: 25 minutes
Servings: 4
Ingredients:
2 chicken breasts, boneless, skinless and halved
1 cup black olives, pitted
½ cup olive oil
Salt and black pepper to the taste
½ cup mixed parsley, chopped
½ cup rosemary, chopped
Salt and black pepper to the taste
4 garlic cloves, minced
Juice of ½ lime
Directions:
1. In a blender, combine the olives with half of the oil and the rest of the ingredients except the chicken and pulse well.
2. Heat up a pan with the rest of the oil over medium-high heat, add the chicken and brown for 4 minutes on each side.
3. Add the olives mix, and cook for 20 minutes more tossing often.
Nutrition: calories 291, fat 12.9, fiber 8.5, carbs 15.8, protein 34.2

Spiced Chicken Meatballs

Preparation time: 10 minutes
Cooking time: 20 minutes
Servings: 4
Ingredients:
- 1 pound chicken meat, ground
- 1 tablespoon pine nuts, toasted and chopped
- 1 egg, whisked
- 2 teaspoons turmeric powder
- 2 garlic cloves, minced
- Salt and black pepper to the taste
- 1 and ¼ cups heavy cream
- 2 tablespoons olive oil
- ¼ cup parsley, chopped
- 1 tablespoon chives, chopped

Directions:
1. In a bowl, combine the chicken with the pine nuts and the rest of the ingredients except the oil and the cream, stir well and shape medium meatballs out of this mix.
2. Heat up a pan with the oil over medium-high heat, add the meatballs and cook them for 4 minutes on each side.
3. Add the cream, toss gently, cook everything over medium heat for 10 minutes more, divide between plates and serve.

Nutrition: calories 283, fat 9.2, fiber 12.8, carbs 24.4, protein 34.5

Sesame Turkey Mix

Preparation time: 10 minutes
Cooking time: 25 minutes
Servings: 4
Ingredients:
- 2 tablespoons avocado oil
- 1 and ¼ cups chicken stock
- 1 tablespoons sesame seeds, toasted
- Salt and black pepper to the taste
- 1 big turkey breast, skinless, boneless and sliced
- ¼ cup parsley, chopped
- 4 ounces feta cheese, crumbled
- ¼ cup red onion, chopped
- 1 tablespoon lemon juice

Directions:
1. Heat up a pan with the oil over medium-high heat, add the meat and brown for 4 minutes on each side.
2. Add the rest of the ingredients except the cheese and the sesame seeds, bring everything to a simmer and cook over medium heat for 15 minutes.
3. Add the cheese, toss, divide the mix between plates, sprinkle the sesame seeds on top and serve.

Nutrition: calories 283, fat 13.2, fiber 6.8, carbs 19.4, protein 24.5

Cardamom Chicken and Apricot Sauce

Preparation time: 10 minutes

Cooking time: 7 hours
Servings: 4
Ingredients:
- Juice of ½ lemon
- Zest of ½ lemon, grated
- 2 teaspoons cardamom, ground
- Salt and black pepper to the taste
- 2 chicken breasts, skinless, boneless and halved
- 2 tablespoons olive oil
- 2 spring onions, chopped
- 2 tablespoons tomato paste
- 2 garlic cloves, minced
- 1 cup apricot juice
- ½ cup chicken stock
- ¼ cup cilantro, chopped

Directions:
1. In your slow cooker, combine the chicken with the lemon juice, lemon zest and the other ingredients except the cilantro, toss, put the lid on and cook on Low for 7 hours.
2. Divide the mix between plates, sprinkle the cilantro on top and serve.

Nutrition: calories 323, fat 12, fiber 11, carbs 23.8, protein 16.4

Meat Recipes

Rosemary Pork Chops

Preparation time: 10 minutes
Cooking time: 35 minutes
Servings: 4
Ingredients:
- 4 pork loin chops, boneless
- Salt and black pepper to the taste
- 4 garlic cloves, minced
- 1 tablespoon rosemary, chopped
- 1 tablespoon olive oil

Directions:
1. In a roasting pan, combine the pork chops with the rest of the ingredients, toss, and bake at 425 degrees F for 10 minutes.
2. Reduce the heat to 350 degrees F and cook the chops for 25 minutes more.
3. Divide the chops between plates and serve with a side salad.

Nutrition: calories 161, fat 5, fiber 1, carbs 1, protein 25

Pork Chops and Relish

Preparation time: 15 minutes
Cooking time: 14 minutes
Servings: 6
Ingredients:
- 6 pork chops, boneless
- 7 ounces marinated artichoke hearts, chopped and their liquid reserved
- A pinch of salt and black pepper
- 1 teaspoon hot pepper sauce
- 1 and ½ cups tomatoes, cubed
- 1 jalapeno pepper, chopped
- ½ cup roasted bell peppers, chopped
- ½ cup black olives, pitted and sliced

Directions:
1. In a bowl, mix the chops with the pepper sauce, reserved liquid from the artichokes, cover and keep in the fridge for 15 minutes.
2. Heat up a grill over medium-high heat, add the pork chops and cook for 7 minutes on each side.
3. In a bowl, combine the artichokes with the peppers and the remaining ingredients, toss, divide on top of the chops and serve.

Nutrition: calories 215, fat 6, fiber 1, carbs 6, protein 35

Pork Chops and Peach Chutney

Preparation time: 10 minutes
Cooking time: 30 minutes
Servings: 4
Ingredients:
- 4 pork loin chops, boneless
- Salt and black pepper to the taste
- ½ teaspoon garlic powder
- ¼ teaspoon cumin, ground
- ½ teaspoon sage, dried
- Cooking spray
- 1 teaspoon chili powder
- 1 teaspoon oregano, dried

For the chutney:
- ¼ cup shallot, minced
- 1 teaspoon olive oil
- 2 cups peaches, peeled and chopped
- ½ cup red sweet pepper, chopped
- 2 tablespoons jalapeno chili pepper, minced
- 1 tablespoon balsamic vinegar
- ½ teaspoon cinnamon powder
- 2 tablespoons cilantro, chopped

Directions:
1. Heat up a pan with the olive oil over medium heat, add the shallot and sauté for 5 minutes.
2. Add the sweet pepper, peaches, chili pepper, vinegar, cinnamon and the cilantro, stir, simmer for 10 minutes and take off the heat.
3. Meanwhile, in a bowl, combine the pork chops with cooking spray, salt, pepper, garlic powder, cumin, sage, oregano and chili powder and rub well.
4. Heat up your grill over medium-high heat, add pork chops, cook for 6-7 minutes on each side, divide between plates and serve with the chutney on top.

Nutrition: calories 297, fat 10, fiber 2, carbs 13, protein 38

Glazed Pork Chops

Preparation time: 10 minutes
Cooking time: 20 minutes
Servings: 4
Ingredients:
- ¼ cup apricot preserves
- 4 pork chops, boneless
- 1 tablespoon thyme, chopped
- ½ teaspoon cinnamon powder
- 2 tablespoons olive oil

Directions:
1. Heat up a pan with the oil over medium-high heat, add the apricot preserves and cinnamon, whisk, bring to a simmer, cook for 10 minutes and take off the heat.
2. Heat up your grill over medium-high heat, brush the pork chops with some of the apricot glaze, place them on the grill and cook for 10 minutes.
3. Flip the chops, brush them with more apricot glaze, cook for 10 minutes more and divide between plates.
4. Sprinkle the thyme on top and serve.

Nutrition: calories 225, fat 11, fiber 0, carbs 6, protein 23

Pork Chops and Cherries Mix

Preparation time: 10 minutes
Cooking time: 12 minutes
Servings: 4
Ingredients:
- 4 pork chops, boneless
- Salt and black pepper to the taste
- ½ cup cranberry juice
- 1 and ½ teaspoons spicy mustard

- ½ cup dark cherries, pitted and halved
- Cooking spray

Directions:
1. Heat up a pan greased with the cooking spray over medium-high heat, add the pork chops, cook them for 5 minutes on each side and divide between plates.
2. Heat up the same pan over medium heat, add the cranberry juice and the rest of the ingredients, whisk, bring to a simmer, cook for 2 minutes, drizzle over the pork chops and serve.

Nutrition: calories 262, fat 8, fiber 1, carbs 16, protein 30

Baked Pork Chops

Preparation time: 10 minutes
Cooking time: 30 minutes
Servings: 4
Ingredients:
- 4 pork loin chops, boneless
- A pinch of salt and black pepper
- 1 tablespoon sweet paprika
- 2 tablespoons Dijon mustard
- Cooking spray

Directions:
1. In a bowl, mix the pork chops with salt, pepper, paprika and the mustard and rub well.
2. Grease a baking sheet with cooking spray, add the pork chops, cover with tin foil, introduce in the oven and bake at 400 degrees F for 30 minutes.
3. Divide the pork chops between plates and serve with a side salad.

Nutrition: calories 167, fat 5, fiber 0, carbs 2, protein 25

Pork Chops with Veggies

Preparation time: 10 minutes
Cooking time: 30 minutes
Servings: 4
Ingredients:
- 4 pork loin chops, boneless
- 1 teaspoon Italian seasoning
- 1 zucchini, sliced
- 1 yellow squash, cubed
- 1 cup cherry tomatoes, halved
- ½ teaspoon oregano, dried
- Salt and black pepper to the taste
- 1 tablespoon olive oil
- 3 garlic cloves, minced
- ¼ cup kalamata olives, pitted and halved
- Juice of 1 lime
- ¼ cup feta cheese, crumbled

Directions:
1. In a roasting pan, combine the pork chops with salt, pepper, seasoning and the rest of the ingredients except the cheese, toss a bit, put the lid on and bake at 360 degrees F for 30 minutes.
2. Divide the mix between plates, sprinkle the cheese on top and serve.

Nutrition: calories 230, fat 9, fiber 2, carbs 9, protein 28

Pork Chops and Herbed Tomato Sauce

Preparation time: 10 minutes
Cooking time: 10 minutes
Servings: 4
Ingredients:
- 4 pork loin chops, boneless
- 6 tomatoes, peeled and crushed
- 3 tablespoons parsley, chopped
- 2 tablespoons olive oil
- ¼ cup kalamata olives, pitted and halved
- 1 yellow onion, chopped
- 1 garlic clove, minced

Directions:
1. Heat up a pan with the oil over medium heat, add the pork chops, cook them for 3 minutes on each side and divide between plates.
2. Heat up the same pan again over medium heat, add the tomatoes, parsley and the rest of the ingredients, whisk, simmer for 4 minutes, drizzle over the chops and serve.

Nutrition: calories 334, fat 17, fiber 2, carbs 12, protein 34

Roasted Lamb Chops

Preparation time: 10 minutes
Cooking time: 27 minutes
Servings: 4
Ingredients:
- 4 lamb chops
- ½ cup basil leaves, chopped
- ½ cup mint leaves, chopped
- 1 tablespoon rosemary, chopped
- 2 garlic cloves, minced
- 2 tablespoons olive oil
- 1 eggplant, cubed
- 2 zucchinis, cubed
- 1 yellow bell pepper, roughly chopped
- 2 ounces feta cheese, crumbled
- 8 ounces cherry tomatoes, halved

Directions:
1. In a roasting pan, combine the pork chops with the basil, mint, rosemary and the rest of the ingredients, cover with tin foil, introduce in the oven and bake at 400 degrees F for 27 minutes.
2. Divide the mix between plates and serve.

Nutrition: calories 334, fat 17, fiber 7, carbs 18, protein 24

Lemon Leg of Lamb Mix

Preparation time: 10 minutes
Cooking time: 40 minutes
Servings: 4
Ingredients:
- 3 pound leg of lamb, boneless
- 2 cups goat cheese, crumbled
- 2 garlic cloves, minced

- 2 teaspoons lemon zest, grated
- 1 tablespoon olive oil
- ½ teaspoon thyme, chopped
- 1 bunch watercress
- 1 tablespoon lemon juice

Directions:
1. Grease a roasting pan with the oil, add the leg of lamb, also add the rest of the ingredients except the goat cheese, introduce in the oven and bake at 425 degrees F for 30 minutes.
2. Add the cheese, toss, bake for 10 minutes more, cool down, slice and serve.

Nutrition: calories 680, fat 55, fiber 1, carbs 4, protein 43

Pork and Chestnuts Mix

Preparation time: 2 hours
Cooking time: 0 minutes
Servings: 6
Ingredients:
- 1 and ½ cups brown rice, already cooked
- 2 cups pork roast, already cooked and shredded
- 3 ounces water chestnuts, drained and sliced
- ½ cup sour cream
- A pinch of salt and white pepper

Directions:
1. In a bowl, mix the rice with the roast and the other ingredients, toss and keep in the fridge for 2 hours before serving.

Nutrition: calories 294, fat 17, fiber 8, carbs 16, protein 23.5

Pork and Sour Cream Mix

Preparation time: 10 minutes
Cooking time: 40 minutes
Servings: 4
Ingredients:
- 1 and ½ pounds pork meat, boneless and cubed
- 1 red onion, chopped
- 1 tablespoon avocado oil
- 1 garlic clove, minced
- ½ cup chicken stock
- 2 tablespoons hot paprika
- Salt and black pepper to the taste
- 1 and ½ cups sour cream
- 1 tablespoon cilantro, chopped

Directions:
1. Heat up a pot with the oil over medium heat, add the pork and brown for 5 minutes.
2. Add the onion and the garlic and cook for 5 minutes more.
3. Add the rest of the ingredients except the cilantro, bring to a simmer and cook over medium heat for 30 minutes.
4. Add the cilantro, toss, divide between plates and serve.

Nutrition: calories 300, fat 9.5, fiber 4.5, carbs 15.5, protein 22

Grilled Pork Chops and Mango Mix

Preparation time: 10 minutes
Cooking time: 22 minutes
Servings: 4
Ingredients:
- 4 pork loin chops, boneless
- 2 tablespoons olive oil
- 2 spring onions, chopped
- 2 garlic cloves, minced
- 2 mangos, peeled and cubed
- 1 teaspoon sweet paprika
- Salt and black pepper to the taste
- ½ teaspoon oregano, dried

Directions:
1. Heat up a pan with the oil over medium-high heat, add the pork chops and brown for 2 minutes on each side.
2. Add the onions and the garlic and brown for 3 minutes more.
3. Add the rest of the ingredients and cook everything for 15 minutes stirring from time to time.
4. Divide the mix between plates and serve.

Nutrition: calories 304, fat 14, fiber 5.6, carbs 12.5, protein 24

Pork and Peas

Preparation time: 10 minutes
Cooking time: 20 minutes
Servings: 4
Ingredients:
- 4 ounces snow peas
- 2 tablespoons avocado oil
- 1 pound pork loin, boneless and cubed
- ¾ cup beef stock
- ½ cup red onion, chopped
- Salt and white pepper to the taste

Directions:
1. Heat up a pan with the oil over medium-high heat, add the pork and brown for 5 minutes.
2. Add the peas and the rest of the ingredients, toss, bring to a simmer and cook over medium heat for 15 minutes.
3. Divide the mix between plates and serve right away.

Nutrition: calories 332, fat 16.5, fiber 10.3, carbs 20.7, protein 26.5

Lime Cumin Pork

Preparation time: 10 minutes
Cooking time: 45 minutes
Servings: 4
Ingredients:
- 1 red onion, chopped
- 1 tablespoon olive oil
- 1 and ½ teaspoons ginger, grated
- 3 garlic cloves, chopped
- Salt and black pepper to the taste
- 2 teaspoons cumin, ground
- 1 and ½ pounds pork meat, roughly cubed
- 2 cups chicken stock

- 2 tablespoons lime juice

Directions:

4. Heat up a pot with the oil over medium heat, add the meat and brown for 5 minutes.
5. Add the onion and garlic and cook for 5 minutes more.
6. Add the rest of the ingredients, bring to a simmer and cook over medium heat for 35 minutes.
7. Divide between plates and serve.

Nutrition: calories 292, fat 16.5, fiber 9.3, carbs 10.7, protein 14.5

Thyme Pork and Pearl Onions

Preparation time: 10 minutes
Cooking time: 45 minutes
Servings: 4
Ingredients:

- 2 pounds pork loin roast, boneless and cubed
- 2 tablespoons olive oil
- Salt and black pepper to the taste
- 1 cup tomato sauce
- 2 garlic cloves, minced
- 1 teaspoon thyme, chopped
- ¾ pound pearl onions, peeled

Directions:

1. In a roasting pan, combine the pork with the oil and the rest of the ingredients, toss, introduce in the oven and bake at 380 degrees F for 45 minutes.
2. Divide the mix between plates and serve.

Nutrition: calories 273, fat 15, fiber 11.6, carbs 16.9, protein 18.8

Tomatoes and Carrots Pork Mix

Preparation time: 10 minutes
Cooking time: 7 hours
Servings: 4
Ingredients:

- 2 tablespoons olive oil
- ½ cup chicken stock
- 1 tablespoon ginger, grated
- Salt and black pepper to the taste
- 2 and ½ pounds pork stew meat, roughly cubed
- 2 cups tomatoes, chopped
- 4 ounces carrots, chopped
- 1 tablespoon cilantro, chopped

Directions:

3. In your slow cooker, combine the oil with the stock, ginger and the rest of the ingredients, put the lid on and cook on Low for 7 hours.
4. Divide the mix between plates and serve.

Nutrition: calories 303, fat 15, fiber 8.6, carbs 14.9, protein 10.8

Pork, Greens and Corn

Preparation time: 10 minutes
Cooking time: 0 minutes
Servings: 4
Ingredients:

- 1 red chili, chopped
- 2 tablespoons balsamic vinegar

- 1 tablespoon lime juice
- 1 teaspoon olive oil
- 4 ounces mixed salad greens
- 2 ounces corn
- 1 green bell pepper, cut into strips
- 4 ounces pork stew meat, cooked and cut in thin strips

Directions:

1. In a bowl, combine the pork with the bell pepper and the rest of the ingredients, toss and keep in the fridge for 10 minutes before serving.
2. Divide the mix between plates and serve.

Nutrition: calories 285, fat 14.6, fiber 10.6, carbs 23.1, protein 13.9

Balsamic Ground Lamb

Preparation time: 5 minutes
Cooking time: 12 minutes
Servings: 4
Ingredients:

- Salt and black pepper to the taste
- 2 tablespoons olive oil
- 6 scallions, chopped
- 2 tablespoons ginger, grated
- 2 garlic cloves, minced
- 1 pound lamb stew, ground
- 1 tablespoon chili paste
- 2 tablespoons balsamic vinegar
- ¼ cup chicken stock
- ¼ cup dill, chopped

Directions:

1. Heat up a pan with the oil over medium high-heat, add the scallions, stir and sauté for 3 minutes.
2. Add the meat and brown for 3 minutes more.
3. Add the rest of the ingredients, toss, cook for 6 minutes more, divide into bowls and serve.

Nutrition: calories 303, fat 13.4, fiber 9.4, carbs 15.2, protein 19.2

Oregano and Pesto Lamb

Preparation time: 10 minutes
Cooking time: 25 minutes
Servings: 4
Ingredients:

- 2 pounds pork shoulder, boneless and cubed
- ¼ cup olive oil
- 2 teaspoons oregano, dried
- ¼ cup lemon juice
- 3 garlic cloves, minced
- 2 teaspoons basil pesto
- Salt and black pepper to the taste

Directions:

1. Heat up a pan with the oil over medium-high heat, add the pork and brown for 5 minutes.
2. Add the rest of the ingredients, cook for 20 minutes more, tossing the mix from time to time, divide between plates and serve.

Nutrition: calories 297, fat 14.5, fiber 9.3, carbs 16.8, protein 22.2

Orange Lamb and Potatoes

Preparation time: 10 minutes
Cooking time: 7 hours
Servings: 4
Ingredients:
- 1 pound small potatoes, peeled and cubed
- 2 cups stewed tomatoes, drained
- Zest and juice of 1 orange
- 4 garlic cloves, minced
- 3 and ½ pounds leg of lamb, boneless and cubed
- Salt and black pepper to the taste
- ½ cup basil, chopped

Directions:
1. In your slow cooker, combine the lamb with the potatoes and the rest of the ingredients, toss, put the lid on and cook on Low for 7 hours.
2. Divide the mix between plates and serve hot.
Nutrition: calories 287, fat 9.5, fiber 7.3, carbs 14.8, protein 18.2

Lamb and Zucchini Mix

Preparation time: 10 minutes
Cooking time: 4 hours
Servings: 4
Ingredients:
- 2 pounds lamb stew meat, cubed
- 1 and ½ tablespoons avocado oil
- 3 zucchinis, sliced
- 1 brown onion, chopped
- 3 garlic cloves, minced
- 1 tablespoon thyme, dried
- 2 teaspoons sage, dried
- 1 cup chicken stock
- 2 tablespoons tomato paste

Directions:
1. In a slow cooker, combine the lamb with the oil, zucchinis and the rest of the ingredients, toss, put the lid on and cook on High for 4 hours.
2. Divide the mix between plates and serve right away.
Nutrition: calories 272, fat 14.5, fiber 10.1, carbs 20.3, protein 13.3

Pork and Sage Couscous

Preparation time: 10 minutes
Cooking time: 7 hours
Servings: 4
Ingredients:
- 2 pounds pork loin boneless and sliced
- ¾ cup veggie stock
- 2 tablespoons olive oil
- ½ tablespoon chili powder
- 2 teaspoon sage, dried
- ½ tablespoon garlic powder
- Salt and black pepper to the taste
- 2 cups couscous, cooked

Directions:

1. In a slow cooker, combine the pork with the stock, the oil and the other ingredients except the couscous, put the lid on and cook on Low for 7 hours.
2. Divide the mix between plates, add the couscous on the side, sprinkle the sage on top and serve.
Nutrition: calories 272, fat 14.5, fiber 9.1, carbs 16.3, protein 14.3

Roasted Basil Pork

Preparation time: 10 minutes
Cooking time: 3 hours
Servings: 6
Ingredients:
- 3 tablespoons garlic, minced
- 1 tablespoon sweet paprika
- 1 tablespoon basil, chopped
- 3 tablespoons olive oil
- 4 pounds pork shoulder
- Salt and black pepper to the taste

Directions:
1. In a roasting pan, combine the pork with the garlic and the other ingredients, toss and bake at 365 degrees F and bake for 3 hours.
2. Take pork shoulder out of the oven, slice, divide between plates and serve with a side salad.
Nutrition: calories 303, fat 14, fiber 14.1, carbs 20.2, protein 17.2

Fennel Pork

Preparation time: 10 minutes
Cooking time: 2 hours
Servings: 4
Ingredients:
- 2 pork loin roast, trimmed, and boneless
- Salt and black pepper to the taste
- 3 garlic cloves, minced
- 2 teaspoons fennel, ground
- 1 tablespoon fennel seeds
- 2 teaspoons red pepper, crushed
- ¼ cup olive oil

Directions:
1. In a roasting pan, combine the pork with salt, pepper and the rest of the ingredients, toss, introduce in the oven and bake at 380 degrees F for 2 hours.
2. Slice the roast, divide between plates and serve with a side salad.
Nutrition: calories 300, fat 4, fiber 2, carbs 6, protein 15

Lamb and Sweet Onion Sauce

Preparation time: 10 minutes
Cooking time: 40 minutes
Servings: 4
Ingredients:
- 2 pounds lamb meat, cubed
- 1 tablespoon sweet paprika
- Salt and black pepper to the taste
- 1 and ½ cups veggie stock

- 4 garlic cloves, minced
- 2 tablespoons olive oil
- 1 pound sweet onion, chopped
- 1 cup balsamic vinegar

Directions:
1.   Heat up a pot with the oil over medium heat, add the onion, vinegar, salt and pepper, stir and cook for 10 minutes.
2.   Add the meat and the rest of the ingredients, toss, bring to a simmer and cook over medium heat for 30 minutes.
3.   Divide the mix between plates and serve.
Nutrition: calories 303, fat 12.3, fiber 7.1, carbs 15.2, protein 17.0

Cheddar Lamb and Zucchinis

Preparation time: 10 minutes
Cooking time: 30 minutes
Servings: 4
Ingredients:
- 1 pound lamb meat, cubed
- 1 tablespoon avocado oil
- 2 cups zucchinis, chopped
- ½ cup red onion, chopped
- Salt and black pepper to the taste
- 15 ounces canned roasted tomatoes, crushed
- ¾ cup cheddar cheese, shredded

Directions:
1.   Heat up a pan with the oil over medium-high heat, add the meat and the onion and brown for 5 minutes.
2.   Add the rest of the ingredients except the cheese, bring to a simmer and cook over medium heat for 20 minutes.
3.   Add the cheese, cook everything for 5 minutes more, divide between plates and serve.
Nutrition: calories 306, fat 16.4, fiber 12.3, carbs 15.5, protein 18.5

Pork and Mustard Shallots Mix

Preparation time: 10 minutes
Cooking time: 25 minutes
Servings: 4
Ingredients:
- 3 shallots, chopped
- 1 pound pork loin, cut into strips
- ½ cup veggie stock
- 2 tablespoons olive oil
- A pinch of salt and black pepper
- 2 teaspoons mustard
- 1 tablespoon parsley, chopped

Directions:
4   Heat up a pan with the oil over medium-high heat, add the shallots and sauté for 5 minutes.
5   Add the meat and cook for 10 minutes tossing it often.
6   Add the rest of the ingredients, toss, cook for 10 minutes more, divide between plates and serve right away.

Nutrition: calories 296, fat 12.4, fiber 9.3, carbs 13.5, protein 22.5

Creamy Pork and Turnips Mix

Preparation time: 10 minutes
Cooking time: 1 hour and 20 minutes
Servings: 4
Ingredients:
- 2 pounds pork loin, sliced
- 2 tablespoons olive oil
- 3 turnips, chopped
- 1 teaspoon black peppercorns, crushed
- 2 red onions, chopped
- 2 cups Greek yogurt
- 1 teaspoon mustard
- Salt and black pepper to the taste

Directions:
1.   Heat up a pan with the oil over medium-high heat, add the meat, brown for 4 minutes on each side and transfer to a bowl.
2.   Heat up the pan again over medium heat, add the onions, turnips and peppercorns and sauté for 5 minutes.
3.   Return the meat, also add the rest of the ingredients, toss, introduce the pan in the oven and bake at 370 degrees F for 1 hour.
4.   Divide everything between plates and serve.
Nutrition: calories 217, fat 7.4, fiber 10.3, carbs 20.8, protein 15.4

Ground Lamb Pan

Preparation time: 10 minutes
Cooking time: 20 minutes
Servings: 4
Ingredients:
- Zest and juice of 2 limes
- 1 and ½ pounds lamb, ground
- 2 garlic cloves, minced
- 2 tablespoons olive oil
- Salt and black pepper to the taste
- 1 pint cherry tomatoes, halved
- 1 small red onion, chopped
- 2 tablespoons tomato paste
- 1 tablespoon rosemary, chopped

Directions:
1.   Heat up a pan with the oil over medium-high heat, add the meat and the garlic and sauté for 5 minutes.
2.   Add the rest of the ingredients, toss, cook for 15 minutes more, divide into bowls and serve.
Nutrition: calories 287, fat 9.4, fiber 10.3, carbs 20.5, protein 15.4

Pork Salad

Preparation time: 10 minutes
Cooking time: 10 minutes
Servings: 4
Ingredients:
- 1 pound pork loin, cut into strips
- 3 scallions, chopped

- 1 cucumber, sliced
- 1 red chili, sliced
- 1 tablespoon coriander leaves, chopped
- 2 ounces walnuts, chopped
- 2 tablespoons olive oil
- Salt and black pepper to the taste
- Juice of 1 lime
- 1 garlic clove, minced

Directions:
1. Heat up a pan with half of the oil over medium-high heat, add the meat, cook for 5 minutes on each side and transfer to a bowl.
2. Add the rest of the ingredients to the bowl as well, toss and serve.
Nutrition: calories 267, fat 13.3, fiber 8.2, carbs 15.2, protein 17.6

Nutmeg Lamb Mix

Preparation time: 10 minutes
Cooking time: 30 minutes
Servings: 6
Ingredients:
- 1 red onion, chopped
- 1 tablespoon olive oil
- 1 garlic clove, minced
- 1 pound lamb meat, cubed
- ¾ cup celery, chopped
- Salt and black pepper to the taste
- 29 ounces canned tomatoes, drained and chopped
- 1 cup veggie stock
- ½ teaspoon nutmeg, ground
- 2 teaspoons parsley, chopped

Directions:
4. Heat up a pan with the oil over medium heat, add the onion and the garlic and sauté for 5 minutes.
5. Add the meat and brown for 5 minutes more.
6. Add the rest of the ingredients, bring to a simmer and cook over medium heat for 20 minutes.
7. Divide everything between plates and serve.
Nutrition: calories 284, fat 13.3, fiber 8.2, carbs 14.5, protein 17.6

Turmeric Pork and Parsnips

Preparation time: 10 minutes
Cooking time: 1 hour and 40 minutes
Servings: 8
Ingredients:
- 1 pound pork loin, sliced
- 2 tablespoons olive oil
- 3 parsnips, sliced
- 1 red onion, chopped
- Salt and black pepper to the taste
- 3 garlic cloves, chopped
- 2 cups veggie stock
- 2 tablespoons tomato paste
- 2 teaspoons turmeric powder
- 1 teaspoon oregano, dried
- 2 tablespoons parsley, chopped

Directions:
4. Heat up a pot with the oil over medium-high heat, add the meat, onion and garlic and brown for 8 minutes.
5. Add the rest of the ingredients, introduce the pan in the oven and bake at 380 degrees F for 1 hour and 20 minutes.
6. Divide everything between plates and serve.
Nutrition: calories 303, fat 23.7, fiber 9.4, carbs 22.8, protein 19.4

Lamb and Wine Sauce

Preparation time: 10 minutes
Cooking time: 2 hours and 40 minutes
Servings: 4
Ingredients:
- 2 tablespoons olive oil
- 2 pounds leg of lamb, trimmed and sliced
- 3 garlic cloves, chopped
- 2 yellow onions, chopped
- 3 cups veggie stock
- 2 cups dry red wine
- 2 tablespoons tomato paste
- 4 tablespoons avocado oil
- 1 teaspoon thyme, chopped
- Salt and black pepper to the taste

Directions:
1. Heat up a pan with the oil over medium-high heat, add the meat, brown for 5 minutes on each side and transfer to a roasting pan.
2. Heat up the pan again over medium heat, add the avocado oil, add the onions and garlic and sauté for 5 minutes.
3. Add the remaining ingredients, stir, bring to a simmer and cook for 10 minutes.
4. Pour the sauce over the meat, introduce the pan in the oven and bake at 370 degrees F for 2 hours and 20 minutes.
5. Divide everything between plates and serve.
Nutrition: calories 273, fat 21, fiber 11.1, carbs 16.2, protein 18.3

Sweet Chili Lamb

Preparation time: 10 minutes
Cooking time: 25 minutes
Servings: 4
Ingredients:
- 1 tablespoon olive oil
- 1 pound lamb stew meat, cubed
- ½ cup sweet chili sauce
- 1 cup carrot, chopped
- ½ cup veggie stock
- 1 tablespoon cilantro, chopped
- Salt and black pepper to the taste

Directions:
1. Heat up a pan with the oil over medium-high heat, add the lamb and brown for 5 minutes.
2. Add the rest of the ingredients, bring to a simmer and cook over medium heat for 20 minutes more.

3.   Divide everything between plates and serve.
Nutrition: calories 287, fat 21.1, fiber 11.8, carbs 25.1, protein 18.9

Italian Pork and Mushrooms

Preparation time: 10 minutes
Cooking time: 7 hours
Servings: 4
Ingredients:
- 2 pounds pork stew meat, cubed
- Salt and black pepper to the taste
- 2 cups veggie stock
- 2 tablespoons olive oil
- 1 yellow onion, chopped
- 2 tablespoons thyme, chopped
- 4 garlic cloves, minced
- 1 pound white mushrooms, chopped
- 2 cups tomatoes, crushed
- ½ cup parsley, chopped

Directions:
1.   In your slow cooker, combine meat with salt, pepper, the stock and the rest of the ingredients, put the lid on and cook on Low for 7 hours.
2.   Divide the mix between plates and serve right away.
Nutrition: calories 328, fat 16.7, fiber 9.5, carbs 11.6, protein 15.7

Lamb and Dill Apples

Preparation time: 10 minutes
Cooking time: 25 minutes
Servings: 4
Ingredients:
- 3 green apples, cored, peeled and cubed
- Juice of 1 lemon
- 1 pound lamb stew meat, cubed
- 1 small bunch dill, chopped
- 3 ounces heavy cream
- 2 tablespoon olive oil
- Salt and black pepper to the taste

Directions:
1.   Heat up a pan with the oil over medium-high heat, add the lamb and brown for 5 minutes.
2.   Add the rest of the ingredients, bring to a simmer and cook over medium heat for 20 minutes.
3.   Divide the mix between plates and serve.
Nutrition: calories 328, fat 16.7, fiber 10.5, carbs 21.6, protein 14.7

Pork Chops and Tarragon Sauce

Preparation time: 10 minutes
Cooking time: 28 minutes
Servings: 4
Ingredients:
- 4 pork chops
- Salt and black pepper to the taste
- 2 tablespoons avocado oil
- ½ cup tomato puree
- 1 tablespoon Italian seasoning
- 1 tablespoon tarragon, chopped

Directions:
1.   Heat up a pan with the avocado oil over medium high heat, add the pork chops and brown for 4 minutes on each side.
2.   Add the rest of the ingredients, introduce the pan in the oven and cook at 400 degrees F for 20 minutes.
3.   Divide everything between plates and serve.
Nutrition: calories 219, fat 18, fiber 10.3, carbs 11.5, protein 12.4

Chili Pork Meatballs

Preparation time: 10 minutes
Cooking time: 20 minutes
Servings: 4
Ingredients:
- 1 pound pork meat, ground
- ½ cup parsley, chopped
- 1 cup yellow onion, chopped
- 4 garlic cloves, minced
- 1 tablespoon ginger, grated
- 1 Thai chili, chopped
- 2 tablespoons olive oil
- 1 cup veggie stock
- 2 tablespoons sweet paprika

Directions:
1.   In a bowl, mix the pork with the other ingredients except the oil, stock and paprika, stir well and shape medium meatballs out of this mix.
2.   Heat up a pan with the oil over medium-high heat, add the meatballs and cook for 4 minutes on each side.
3.   Add the stock and the paprika, toss gently, simmer everything over medium heat for 12 minutes more, divide into bowls and serve.
Nutrition: calories 224, fat 18, fiber 9.3, carbs 11.5, protein 14.4

Lamb and Peanuts Mix

Preparation time: 10 minutes
Cooking time: 20 minutes
Servings: 4
Ingredients:
- 2 tablespoons lime juice
- 1 tablespoon balsamic vinegar
- 5 garlic cloves, minced
- 2 tablespoons olive oil
- Salt and black pepper to the taste
- 1 and ½ pound lamb meat, cubed
- 3 tablespoons peanuts, toasted and chopped
- 2 scallions, chopped

Directions:
1.   Heat up a pan with the oil over medium-high heat, add the meat, and cook for 4 minutes on each side.
2.   Add the scallions and the garlic and sauté for 2 minutes more.
3.   Add the rest of the ingredients, toss cook for 10 minutes more, divide between plates and serve right away.

Nutrition: calories 300, fat 14.5, fiber 9.1, carbs 15.7, protein 17.5

Lamb and Green Onions Mix

Preparation time: 10 minutes
Cooking time: 25 minutes
Servings: 4
Ingredients:
- 1 and ½ pounds lamb, cubed
- 2 garlic cloves, minced
- 2 tablespoons olive oil
- Salt and black pepper to the taste
- ½ cup veggie stock
- ½ teaspoon saffron powder
- ¼ teaspoon cumin, ground
- 4 green onions, sliced

Directions:
1. Heat up a pan with the oil over medium-high heat, add the garlic, green onions, saffron and cumin, stir and sauté for 5 minutes.
2. Add the meat and brown it for 5 minutes more.
3. Add salt, pepper and the stock, toss, bring to a simmer and cook over medium heat for 15 minutes more.
4. Divide everything between plates and serve right away.

Nutrition: calories 292, fat 13.2, fiber 9.6, carbs 13.3, protein 14.2

Pork Chops and Peppercorns Mix

Preparation time: 10 minutes
Cooking time: 20 minutes
Servings: 4
Ingredients:
- 1 cup red onion, sliced
- 1 tablespoon black peppercorns, crushed
- ¼ cup veggie stock
- 5 garlic cloves, minced
- A pinch of salt and black pepper
- 2 tablespoons olive oil
- 4 pork chops

Directions:
1. Heat up a pan with the oil over medium-high heat, add the pork chops and brown for 4 minutes on each side.
2. Add the onion and the garlic and cook for 2 minutes more.
3. Add the rest of the ingredients, cook everything for 10 minutes, tossing the mix from time to time, divide between plates and serve.

Nutrition: calories 232, fat 9.2, fiber 5.6, carbs 13.3, protein 24.2

Lamb and Barley Mix

Preparation time: 10 minutes
Cooking time: 8 hours and 10 minutes
Servings: 4
Ingredients:
- 2 tablespoons olive oil

- 1 cup barley soaked overnight, drained and rinsed
- 1 pound lamb meat, cubed
- 1 red onion, chopped
- 4 garlic cloves, minced
- 3 carrots, chopped
- 6 tablespoons dill, chopped
- 2 tablespoons tomato paste
- 3 cups veggie stock
- A pinch of salt and black pepper

Directions:
1. Heat up a pan with the oil over medium-high heat, add the meat, brown for 5 minutes on each side and transfer to your slow cooker.
2. Add the barley and the rest of the ingredients, put the lid on and cook on Low for 8 hours.
3. Divide everything between plates and serve.

Nutrition: calories 292, fat 12.1, fiber 8.7, carbs 16.7, protein 7.2

Pork and Cabbage Mix

Preparation time: 10 minutes
Cooking time: 8 hours and 10 minutes
Servings: 4
Ingredients:
- 2 pounds pork stew meat, roughly cubed
- 1 and ½ cups veggie stock
- 2 red onions, sliced
- 2 tablespoons olive oil
- 2 garlic cloves, minced
- 1 tablespoon sweet paprika
- 1 green cabbage head, shredded
- ½ cup tomato sauce
- Salt and black pepper to the taste
- ¼ cup dill, chopped

Directions:
1. Heat up a pan with the oil over medium-high heat, add the meat, brown for 5 minutes on each side and transfer to a slow cooker.
2. Add the onions, the stock and the rest of the ingredients, put the lid on and cook on Low for 8 hours.
3. Divide the mix between plates and serve right away.

Nutrition: calories 299, fat 14.2, fiber 10.7, carbs 16.3, protein 15.4

Lamb and Rice

Preparation time: 10 minutes
Cooking time: 1 hour and 10 minutes
Servings: 4
Ingredients:
- 1 tablespoon lime juice
- 1 yellow onion, chopped
- 1 pound lamb, cubed
- 1 ounce avocado oil
- 2 garlic cloves, minced
- Salt and black pepper to the taste
- 2 cups veggie stock
- 1 cup brown rice

- A handful parsley, chopped

Directions:
1. Heat up a pan with the avocado oil over medium-high heat, add the onion, stir and sauté for 5 minutes.
2. Add the meat and brown for 5 minutes more.
3. Add the rest of the ingredients except the parsley, bring to a simmer and cook over medium heat for 1 hour.
4. Add the parsley, toss, divide everything between plates and serve.

Nutrition: calories 302, fat 13.2, fiber 10.7, carbs 15.7, protein 14.3

Lamb and Raisins

Preparation time: 10 minutes
Cooking time: 30 minutes
Servings: 4
Ingredients:
- 1 cup raisins
- 1 and ½ pounds lamb, cubed
- 1 tablespoon olive oil
- 1 garlic clove, minced
- 1 yellow onion, grated
- 1 tablespoon ginger, grated
- 2 tablespoons orange juice
- A pinch of salt and black pepper
- 1 cup veggie stock

Directions:
1. Heat up a pan with the oil over medium-high heat, add the garlic and the onion and sauté for 5 minutes.
2. Add the lamb and brown for 5 minutes more.
3. Add the rest of the ingredients, bring to a simmer and cook over medium heat for 20 minutes.
4. Divide the mix between plates and serve.

Nutrition: calories 292, fat 13.2, fiber 9.7, carbs 17.7, protein 16.3

Sour Cream Lamb Mix

Preparation time: 10 minutes
Cooking time: 2 hours and 15 minutes
Servings: 4
Ingredients:
- 2 pounds leg of lamb, boneless
- 2 tablespoons mustard
- ½ cup avocado oil
- 2 tablespoons basil, chopped
- 2 tablespoons tomato paste
- 2 garlic cloves, minced
- Salt and black pepper to the taste
- 1 cup white wine
- ½ cup sour cream

Directions:
1. Heat up a pan with the avocado oil over medium-high heat, add the meat and brown it for 6 minutes on each side.
2. Add the rest of the ingredients, introduce the pan in the oven and cook at 370 degrees F for 2 hours.

3. Divide the mix between plates and serve.

Nutrition: calories 312, fat 12.1, fiber 16.4, carbs 21.7, protein 14.2

Garlic Lamb and Peppers

Preparation time: 10 minutes
Cooking time: 1 hour and 30 minutes
Servings: 4
Ingredients:
- 1 red bell pepper, sliced
- 1 green bell pepper, sliced
- 1 yellow bell pepper, sliced
- 2 tablespoons olive oil
- 1/3 cup mint, chopped
- 4 garlic cloves, minced
- ½ cup veggie stock
- 1 and ½ tablespoon lemon juice
- 4 lamb chops
- Salt and black pepper to the taste

Directions:
1. Heat up a pan with the oil over medium-high heat, add the lamb chops and brown for 4 minutes on each side.
2. Add the rest of the ingredients, introduce the pan in the oven and bake at 370 degrees F for 1 hour and 20 minutes.
3. Divide the mix between plates and serve.

Nutrition: calories 300, fat 14.1, fiber 9.4, carbs 15.7, protein 24.2

Lamb and Cauliflower Mix

Preparation time: 10 minutes
Cooking time: 1 hour
Servings: 4
Ingredients:
- 2 pounds lamb meat, roughly cubed
- 2 tablespoons olive oil
- 1 teaspoon garlic, minced
- 1 yellow onion, chopped
- 1 teaspoon rosemary, chopped
- 1 cup veggie stock
- 2 cups cauliflower florets
- 2 tablespoons sweet paprika
- Salt and pepper to the taste

Directions:
1. Heat up a pot with the oil over medium-high heat, add the onion and the garlic and sauté for 5 minutes.
2. Add the meat and brown for 5-6 minutes more.
3. Add the rest of the ingredients, bring to a simmer and cook over medium heat for 50 minutes.
4. Divide the mix between plates and serve away.

Nutrition: calories 336, fat 14.4, fiber 10.8, carbs 21.7, protein 23.2

Allspice Pork Mix

Preparation time: 10 minutes
Cooking time: 8 hours
Servings: 4
Ingredients:

- 2 pounds pork loin, sliced
- 1 tablespoon olive oil
- Salt and white pepper to the taste
- 2 shallots, chopped
- 2 teaspoons whole allspice, ground
- 1 cup veggie stock
- 1 tablespoon tomato paste
- 2 bay leaves

Directions:
4.   In your slow cooker, combine the pork with the oil, salt, pepper and the rest of the ingredients, put the lid on and cook on Low for 8 hours.
5.   Divide the mix between plates and serve right away.

Nutrition: calories 329, fat 14.2, fiber 11.7, carbs 18.3, protein 23.4

Minty Balsamic Lamb

Preparation time: 10 minutes
Cooking time: 11 minutes
Servings: 4
Ingredients:
- 2 red chilies, chopped
- 2 tablespoons balsamic vinegar
- 1 cup mint leaves, chopped
- Salt and black pepper to the taste
- 2 tablespoons olive oil
- 4 lamb fillets
- 1 tablespoon sweet paprika

Directions:
1.   Heat up a pan with half of the oil over medium-high heat, add the chilies, the vinegar and the rest of the ingredients except the lamb, whisk and cook over medium heat for 5 minutes.
2.   Brush the lamb with the rest of the oil, season with salt and black pepper, place on preheated grill and cook over medium heat for 3 minutes on each side.
3.   Divide the lamb between plates, drizzle the minty vinaigrette all over and serve.

Nutrition: calories 312, fat 12.1, fiber 9.1, carbs 17.7, protein 17.2

Tasty Lamb Ribs

Preparation time: 10 minutes
Cooking time: 2 hours
Servings: 4
Ingredients:
- 2 garlic cloves, minced
- ¼ cup shallot, chopped
- 2 tablespoons fish sauce
- ½ cup veggie stock
- 2 tablespoons olive oil
- 1 and ½ tablespoons lemon juice
- 1 tablespoon coriander seeds, ground
- 1 tablespoon ginger, grated
- Salt and black pepper to the taste
- 2 pounds lamb ribs

Directions:

1.   In a roasting pan, combine the lamb with the garlic, shallots and the rest of the ingredients, toss, introduce in the oven at 300 degrees F and cook for 2 hours.
2.   Divide the lamb between plates and serve with a side salad.

Nutrition: calories 293, fat 9.1, fiber 9.6, carbs 16.7, protein 24.2

Cinnamon and Coriander Lamb

Preparation time: 10 minutes
Cooking time: 6 hours
Servings: 4
Ingredients:
- 2 and ½ pounds lamb shoulder, cubed
- 2 tomatoes, chopped
- 1 garlic clove, minced
- 1 tablespoon cinnamon powder
- Salt and black pepper to the taste
- ½ cup veggie stock
- 1 bunch coriander, chopped

Directions:
1.   In your slow cooker, combine the lamb with the tomatoes and the rest of the ingredients, put the lid on and cook on Low for 6 hours.
2.   Divide everything between plates and serve.

Nutrition: calories 352, fat 15.2, fiber 10.7, carbs 18.7, protein 15.3

Lamb and Plums Mix

Preparation time: 5 minutes
Cooking time: 6 hours and 10 minutes
Servings: 4
Ingredients:
- 4 lamb shanks
- 1 red onion, chopped
- 2 tablespoons olive oil
- 1 cup plums, pitted and halved
- 1 tablespoon sweet paprika
- 2 cups chicken stock
- Salt and pepper to the taste

Directions:
1.   Heat up a pan with the oil over medium-high heat, add the lamb, brown for 5 minutes on each side and transfer to your slow cooker.
2.   Add the rest of the ingredients, put the lid on and cook on High for 6 hours.
3.   Divide the mix between plates and serve right away.

Nutrition: calories 293, fat 13.2, fiber 9.7, carbs 15.7, protein 14.3

Rosemary Lamb

Preparation time: 10 minutes
Cooking time: 6 hours
Servings: 4
Ingredients:
- 2 pounds lamb shoulder, cubed
- 1 tablespoon rosemary, chopped
- 3 garlic cloves, minced

- ½ cup lamb stock
- 4 bay leaves
- Salt and black pepper to the taste

Directions:
1. In your slow cooker, combine the lamb with the rosemary and the rest of the ingredients, put the lid on and cook on High for 6 hours.
2. Divide the mix between palates and serve.

Nutrition: calories 292, fat 13.2, fiber 11.6, carbs 18.3, protein 14.2

Lemony Lamb and Potatoes

Preparation time: 10 minutes
Cooking time: 2 hours and 10 minutes
Servings: 4
Ingredients:
- 2 pound lamb meat, cubed
- 2 tablespoons olive oil
- 2 springs rosemary, chopped
- 2 tablespoons parsley, chopped
- 1 tablespoon lemon rind, grated
- 3 garlic cloves, minced
- 2 tablespoons lemon juice
- 2 pounds baby potatoes, scrubbed and halved
- 1 cup veggie stock

Directions:
1. In a roasting pan, combine the meat with the oil and the rest of the ingredients, introduce in the oven and bake at 400 degrees F for 2 hours and 10 minutes.
2. Divide the mix between plates and serve.

Nutrition: calories 302, fat 15.2, fiber 10.6, carbs 23.3, protein 15.2

Lamb and Feta Artichokes

Preparation time: 10 minutes
Cooking time: 8 hours and 5 minutes
Servings: 6
Ingredients:
- 2 pounds lamb shoulder, boneless and roughly cubed
- 2 spring onions, chopped
- 1 tablespoon olive oil
- 3 garlic cloves, minced
- 1 tablespoon lemon juice
- Salt and black pepper to the taste
- 1 and ½ cups veggie stock
- 6 ounces canned artichoke hearts, drained and quartered
- ½ cup feta cheese, crumbled
- 2 tablespoons parsley, chopped

Directions:
1. Heat up a pan with the oil over medium-high heat, add the lamb, brown 5 minutes and transfer to your slow cooker.
2. Add the rest of the ingredients except the parsley and the cheese, put the lid on and cook on Low for 8 hours.
3. Add the cheese and the parsley, divide the mix between plates and serve.

Nutrition: calories 330, fat 14.5, fiber 14.1, carbs 21.7, protein 17.5

Lamb and Mango Sauce

Preparation time: 10 minutes
Cooking time: 1 hour
Servings: 4
Ingredients:
- 2 cups Greek yogurt
- 1 cup mango, peeled and cubed
- 1 yellow onion, chopped
- 1/3 cup parsley, chopped
- 1 pound lamb, cubed
- ½ teaspoon red pepper flakes
- Salt and black pepper to the taste
- 2 tablespoons olive oil
- ¼ teaspoon cinnamon powder

Directions:
1. Heat up a pan with the oil over medium-high heat, add the meat and brown for 5 minutes.
2. Add the onion and sauté for 5 minutes more.
3. Add the rest of the ingredients, toss, bring to a simmer and cook over medium heat for 45 minutes.
4. Divide everything between plates and serve.

Nutrition: calories 300, fat 15.5, fiber 9.1, carbs 15.7, protein 15.5

Pork Chops with Sweet Peppers and Cabbage

Preparation time: 10 minutes
Cooking time: 23 minutes
Servings: 4
Ingredients:
- 4 pork chops
- 1 teaspoon rosemary, dried
- 2 teaspoons olive oil
- 3 tablespoons wine vinegar
- 2 spring onions, chopped
- ½ green cabbage head, shredded
- 4 sweet peppers, chopped
- Salt and black pepper to the taste

Directions:
1. Heat up a pan with half of the oil over medium-high heat, add spring onions and sauté for 3 minutes.
2. Add the rest of the ingredients except the pork chops and rosemary, stir, simmer for 10 minutes and take off the heat.
3. Rub the pork chops with the rest of the oil, season with salt, pepper and the rosemary, place on preheated grill and cook over medium-high heat for 5 minutes on each side.
4. Divide the chops between plates, add the cabbage and peppers mix on the side and serve.

Nutrition: calories 219, fat 18, fiber 9.3, carbs 16.5, protein 12.4

Greek Lamb And Eggplant

Preparation time: 10 minutes
Cooking time: 1 hour
Servings: 4

Ingredients:
- 4 eggplants, cubed
- 3 tablespoons olive oil
- 2 yellow onions, chopped
- 1 and ½ pounds lamb meat, roughly cubed
- 2 tablespoons tomato paste
- ½ cup parsley, chopped
- 4 garlic cloves, minced
- ½ cup Greek yogurt

Directions:
1. Heat up a pan with the olive oil over medium-high heat, add the onions and garlic and sauté for 4 minutes.
2. Add the meat and brown for 6 minutes.
3. Add the eggplants and the other ingredients except the parsley, bring to a simmer and cook over medium heat for 50 minutes more stirring from time to time.
4. Divide everything between plates and serve.

Nutrition: calories 299, fat 18, fiber 14.3, carbs 21.5, protein 14.4

Pork Kebabs

Preparation time: 10 minutes
Cooking time: 14 minutes
Servings: 6
Ingredients:
- 1 yellow onion, chopped
- 1 pound pork meat, ground
- 3 tablespoons cilantro, chopped
- 1 tablespoon lime juice
- 1 garlic clove, minced
- 2 teaspoon oregano, dried
- Salt and black pepper to the taste
- A drizzle of olive oil

Directions:
1. In a bowl, mix the pork with the other ingredients except the oil, stir well and shape medium kebabs out of this mix.
2. Divide the kebabs on skewers, and brush them with a drizzle of oil.
3. Place the kebabs on your preheated grill and cook over medium heat for 7 minutes on each side.
4. Divide the kebabs between plates and serve with a side salad.

Nutrition: calories 229, fat 14, fiber 8.3, carbs 15.5, protein 12.4

Cilantro Pork and Olives
!

Preparation time: 10 minutes
Cooking time: 20 minutes
Servings: 4
Ingredients:
- 2 pounds pork loin, sliced
- 1 cup black olives, pitted and halved
- 2 tablespoons olive oil
- ½ cup tomato puree
- Salt and black pepper to the taste
- ½ cup mixed cilantro, chopped

- Salt and black pepper to the taste
- 4 garlic cloves, minced
- Juice of 1 lime

Directions:
1. Heat up a pan with the oil over medium-high heat, add the garlic and the meat and brown for 5 minutes.
2. Add the rest of the ingredients, bring to a simmer and cook over medium heat for 15 minutes more.
3. Divide the mix between plates and serve.

Nutrition: calories 249, fat 12, fiber 8.3, carbs 21.5, protein 12.6

Pork and Parsley Sauce

Preparation time: 10 minutes
Cooking time: 20 minutes
Servings: 4
Ingredients:
- 1 pound pork stew meat, cubed
- 1 tablespoon walnuts, chopped
- 1 cup parsley, chopped
- 2 garlic cloves, minced
- Salt and black pepper to the taste
- 2 cups Greek yogurt
- ½ cup olive oil

Directions:
1. In a blender, combine the parsley with garlic, walnuts, yogurt, salt, pepper and half of the oil and pulse well.
2. Heat up a pan with the rest of the oil over medium-high heat, add the meat and cook for 5 minutes.
3. Add the parsley sauce, toss, bring to a simmer and cook over medium heat for 15 minutes more.
4. Divide the mix into bowls and serve.

Nutrition: calories 264, fat 11, fiber 5.4, carbs 20.1, protein 18.5

Pork Tenderloin and Dill Sauce

Preparation time: 10 minutes
Cooking time: 20 minutes
Servings: 4
Ingredients:
- 1 pound pork tenderloin, sliced
- Salt and black pepper to the taste
- 3 tablespoons coriander seeds, ground
- 2 tablespoons olive oil
- 1/3 cup heavy cream
- ½ cup dill, chopped

Directions:
1. Heat up a pan with the oil over medium-high heat, add the meat and brown for 4 minutes on each side.
2. Add the rest of the ingredients, bring to a simmer and cook over medium heat for 12 minutes more.
3. Divide the mix between plates and serve.

Nutrition: calories 320, fat 14.5, fiber 9.1, carbs 13.7, protein 17.5

Lamb and Couscous

Preparation time: 10 minutes
Cooking time: 30 minutes
Servings: 4
Ingredients:
1 and ½ cups couscous
2 tablespoons avocado oil
2 cups chicken stock
1 tablespoon cilantro, chopped
Salt and black pepper to the taste
1 and ½ pound lamb meat, cubed
¼ cup parsley, chopped
4 ounces feta cheese, crumbled
¼ cup spring onions, chopped
Directions:
1.   Heat up a pan with the oil over medium-high heat, add the lamb and brown for 6 minutes.
2.   Add the couscous and brown for 4 minutes more.
3.   Add the rest of the ingredients except the cheese, bring to a simmer and cook over medium heat for 20 minutes more.
4.   Add the cheese, toss, divide the mix between plates and serve.
Nutrition: calories 370, fat 24.5, fiber 11, carbs 16.7, protein 27.5

Pork Meatloaf

Preparation time: 10 minutes
Cooking time: 1 hour and 20 minutes
Servings: 6
Ingredients:
- 1 red onion, chopped
- Cooking spray
- 2 garlic cloves, minced
- 2 pounds pork stew, ground
- 1 cup almond milk
- ¼ cup feta cheese, crumbled
- 2 eggs, whisked
- 1/3 cup kalamata olives, pitted and chopped
- 4 tablespoons oregano, chopped
- Salt and black pepper to the taste
Directions:
1.   In a bowl, mix the meat with the onion, garlic and the other ingredients except the cooking spray, stir well, shape your meatloaf and put it in a loaf pan greased with cooking spray.
2.   Bake the meatloaf at 370 degrees F for 1 hour and 20 minutes.
3.   Serve the meatloaf warm.
Nutrition: calories 350, fat 23, fiber 1, carbs 17, protein 24

Marjoram Pork

Preparation time: 10 minutes
Cooking time: 1 hour
Servings: 4
Ingredients:
- 1 cup marjoram, chopped
- 1 garlic clove, minced

- 1 tablespoons capers, drained
- 2 tablespoons olive oil
- 1 and ½ pounds pork loin, cubed
- 1 cup veggie stock
- Salt and black pepper to the taste
- ½ cup feta cheese, crumbled
Directions:
1.   Heat up a pan with the oil over medium-high heat, add the meat and brown for 5 minutes.
2.   Add the rest of the ingredients except the cheese, toss, bring to a simmer and cook over medium heat for 30 minutes.
3.   Add the cheese, toss gently, divide between plates and serve.
Nutrition: calories 304, fat 14.1, fiber 8.2, carbs 15.9, protein 33.2

Italian Pork Spareribs

Preparation time: 10 minutes
Cooking time: 1 hour and 30 minutes
Servings: 4
Ingredients:
2 pork spareribs
2 teaspoons basil, dried
1 teaspoon rosemary, dried
2 teaspoons smoked paprika
Salt and black pepper to the taste
4 garlic cloves, minced
6 tablespoons sherry vinegar
¼ cup olive oil
Directions:
1.   In a bowl, mix the ribs with the rest of the ingredients, toss and keep in the fridge for 10 minutes.
2.   Heat up your grill over medium-high heat, add the spareribs, cover your grill and cook them for 1 hour and 30 minutes flipping from time to time.
3.   Divide between plates and serve with a side salad.
Nutrition: calories 344, fat 21, fiber 12.2, carbs 19.9, protein 23.2

Pork and Figs Mix

Preparation time: 10 minutes
Cooking time: 40 minutes
Servings: 4
Ingredients:
- 3 tablespoons avocado oil
- 1 and ½ pounds pork stew meat, roughly cubed
- Salt and black pepper to the taste
- 1 cup red onions, chopped
- 1 cup figs, dried and chopped
- 1 tablespoon ginger, grated
- 1 tablespoon garlic, minced
- 1 cup canned tomatoes, crushed
- 2 tablespoons parsley, chopped
Directions:
1.   Heat up a pot with the oil over medium-high heat, add the meat and brown for 5 minutes.
2.   Add the onions and sauté for 5 minutes more.

3.   Add the rest of the ingredients, bring to a simmer and cook over medium heat for 30 minutes more.
4.   Divide the mix between plates and serve.
Nutrition: calories 309, fat 16, fiber 10.4, carbs 21.1, protein 34.2

Pomegranate Pork and Sweet Potatoes

Preparation time: 10 minutes
Cooking time: 50 minutes
Servings: 4
Ingredients:
- 1 and ½ pounds pork meat, cubed
- Salt and black pepper to the taste
- Zest of 1 orange, grated
- 1 teaspoon rosemary, chopped
- 1 cup pomegranate juice
- 2 tablespoons avocado oil
- 2 sweet potatoes, cubed
- 1 cup veggie stock

Directions:
1.   Heat up a pan with the oil over medium-high heat, add the meat and brown for 5 minutes.
2.   Add the rest of the ingredients, bring everything to a simmer and cook over medium heat for 45 minutes more stirring from time to time.
3.   Divide everything between plates and serve.
Nutrition: calories 546, fat 23, fiber 5, carbs 14, protein 24

Vegetable Recipes

Peppers and Lentils Salad

Preparation time: 10 minutes
Cooking time: 0 minutes
Servings: 4
Ingredients:
- 14 ounces canned lentils, drained and rinsed
- 2 spring onions, chopped
- 1 red bell pepper, chopped
- 1 green bell pepper, chopped
- 1 tablespoon fresh lime juice
- 1/3 cup coriander, chopped
- 2 teaspoon balsamic vinegar

Directions:
1. In a salad bowl, combine the lentils with the onions, bell peppers and the rest of the ingredients, toss and serve.
Nutrition: calories 200, fat 2.45, fiber 6.7, carbs 10.5, protein 5.6

Cashews and Red Cabbage Salad

Preparation time: 10 minutes
Cooking time: 0 minutes
Servings: 4
Ingredients:
- 1 pound red cabbage, shredded
- 2 tablespoons coriander, chopped
- ½ cup cashews, halved
- 2 tablespoons olive oil
- 1 tomato, cubed
- A pinch of salt and black pepper
- 1 tablespoon white vinegar

Directions:
1. In a salad bowl, combine the cabbage with the coriander and the rest of the ingredients, toss and serve cold.
Nutrition: calories 210, fat 6.3, fiber 5.2, carbs 5.5, protein 8

Apples and Pomegranate Salad

Preparation time: 10 minutes
Cooking time: 0 minutes
Servings: 4
Ingredients:
- 3 big apples, cored and cubed
- 1 cup pomegranate seeds
- 3 cups baby arugula
- 1 cup walnuts, chopped
- 1 tablespoon olive oil
- 1 teaspoon white sesame seeds
- 2 tablespoons apple cider vinegar
- Salt and black pepper to the taste

Directions:
4 In a bowl, mix the apples with the arugula and the rest of the ingredients, toss and serve cold.
Nutrition: calories 160, fat 4.3, fiber 5.3, carbs 8.7, protein 10

Cranberry Bulgur Mix

Preparation time: 10 minutes
Cooking time: 0 minutes
Servings: 4
Ingredients:
- 1 and ½ cups hot water
- 1 cup bulgur
- Juice of ½ lemon
- 4 tablespoons cilantro, chopped
- ½ cup cranberries, chopped
- 1 and ½ teaspoons curry powder
- ¼ cup green onions, chopped
- ½ cup red bell peppers, chopped
- ½ cup carrots, grated
- 1 tablespoon olive oil
- A pinch of salt and black pepper

Directions:
1. Put bulgur into a bowl, add the water, stir, cover, leave aside for 10 minutes, fluff with a fork and transfer to a bowl.
2. Add the rest of the ingredients, toss, and serve cold.
Nutrition: calories 300, fat 6.4, fiber 6.1, carbs 7.6, protein 13

Chickpeas, Corn and Black Beans Salad

Preparation time: 10 minutes
Cooking time: 0 minutes
Servings: 4
Ingredients:
- 1 and ½ cups canned black beans, drained and rinsed
- ½ teaspoon garlic powder
- 2 teaspoons chili powder
- A pinch of sea salt and black pepper
- 1 and ½ cups canned chickpeas, drained and rinsed
- 1 cup baby spinach
- 1 avocado, pitted, peeled and chopped
- 1 cup corn kernels, chopped
- 2 tablespoons lemon juice
- 1 tablespoon olive oil
- 1 tablespoon apple cider vinegar
- 1 teaspoon chives, chopped

Directions:
1. In a salad bowl, combine the black beans with the garlic powder, chili powder and the rest of the ingredients, toss and serve cold.
Nutrition: calories 300, fat 13.4, fiber 4.1, carbs 8.6, protein 13

Olives and Lentils Salad

Preparation time: 10 minutes
Cooking time: 0 minutes
Servings: 2
Ingredients:
- 1/3 cup canned green lentils, drained and rinsed

- 1 tablespoon olive oil
- 2 cups baby spinach
- 1 cup black olives, pitted and halved
- 2 tablespoons sunflower seeds
- 1 tablespoon Dijon mustard
- 2 tablespoons balsamic vinegar
- 2 tablespoons olive oil

Directions:
4   In a bowl, mix the lentils with the spinach, olives and the rest of the ingredients, toss and serve cold.
Nutrition: calories 279, fat 6.5, fiber 4.5, carbs 9.6, protein 12

Lime Spinach and Chickpeas Salad
Preparation time: 10 minutes
Cooking time: 0 minutes
Servings: 4
Ingredients:
- 16 ounces canned chickpeas, drained and rinsed
- 2 cups baby spinach leaves
- ½ tablespoon lime juice
- 2 tablespoons olive oil
- 1 teaspoon cumin, ground
- A pinch of sea salt and black pepper
- ½ teaspoon chili flakes

Directions:
1.   In a bowl, mix the chickpeas with the spinach and the rest of the ingredients, toss and serve cold.
Nutrition: calories 240, fat 8.2, fiber 5.3, carbs 11.6, protein 12

Minty Olives and Tomatoes Salad
Preparation time: 10 minutes
Cooking time: 0 minutes
Servings: 4
Ingredients:
- 1 cup kalamata olives, pitted and sliced
- 1 cup black olives, pitted and halved
- 1 cup cherry tomatoes, halved
- 4 tomatoes, chopped
- 1 red onion, chopped
- 2 tablespoons oregano, chopped
- 1 tablespoon mint, chopped
- 2 tablespoons balsamic vinegar
- ¼ cup olive oil
- 2 teaspoons Italian herbs, dried
- A pinch of sea salt and black pepper

Directions:
1.   In a salad bowl, mix the olives with the tomatoes and the rest of the ingredients, toss and serve cold.
Nutrition: calories 190, fat 8.1, fiber 5.8, carbs 11.6, protein 4.6

Beans and Cucumber Salad
Preparation time: 10 minutes
Cooking time: 0 minutes
Servings: 4

Ingredients:
- 15 ounces canned great northern beans, drained and rinsed
- 2 tablespoons olive oil
- ½ cup baby arugula
- 1 cup cucumber, sliced
- 1 tablespoon parsley, chopped
- 2 tomatoes, cubed
- A pinch of sea salt and black pepper
- 2 tablespoon balsamic vinegar

Directions:
1.   In a bowl, mix the beans with the cucumber and the rest of the ingredients, toss and serve cold.
Nutrition: calories 233, fat 9, fiber 6.5, carbs 13, protein 8

Tomato And Avocado Salad
Preparation time: 10 minutes
Cooking time: 0 minutes
Servings: 4
Ingredients:
- 1 pound cherry tomatoes, cubed
- 2 avocados, pitted, peeled and cubed
- 1 sweet onion, chopped
- A pinch of sea salt and black pepper
- 2 tablespoons lemon juice
- 1 and ½ tablespoons olive oil
- A handful basil, chopped

Directions:
1.   In a salad bowl, mix the tomatoes with the avocados and the rest of the ingredients, toss and serve right away.
Nutrition: calories 148, fat 7.8, fiber 2.9, carbs 5.4, protein 5.5

Corn and Tomato Salad
Preparation time: 10 minutes
Cooking time: 0 minutes
Servings: 4
Ingredients:
- 2 avocados, pitted, peeled and cubed
- 1 pint mixed cherry tomatoes, halved:
- 2 tablespoons avocado oil
- 1 tablespoon lime juice
- ½ teaspoon lime zest, grated
- A pinch of salt and black pepper
- ¼ cup dill, chopped

Directions:
1.   In a salad bowl, mix the avocados with the tomatoes and the rest of the ingredients, toss and serve cold.
Nutrition: calories 188, fat 7.3, fiber 4.9, carbs 6.4, protein 6.5

Orange and Cucumber Salad
Preparation time: 10 minutes
Cooking time: 0 minutes
Servings: 4
Ingredients:
- 2 cucumbers, sliced

- 1 orange, peeled and cut into segments
- 1 cup cherry tomatoes, halved
- 1 small red onion, chopped
- 3 tablespoons olive oil
- 4 and ½ teaspoons balsamic vinegar
- Salt and black pepper to the taste
- 1 tablespoon lemon juice

Directions:
1. In a bowl, mix the cucumbers with the orange and the rest of the ingredients, toss and serve cold.
Nutrition: calories 102, fat 7.5, fiber 3, carbs 6.1, protein 3.4

Parsley and Corn Salad
Preparation time: 10 minutes
Cooking time: 0 minutes
Servings: 4
Ingredients:
- 1 and ½ teaspoons balsamic vinegar
- 2 tablespoons lime juice
- 2 tablespoons olive oil
- A pinch of sea salt and black pepper
- Black pepper to the taste
- 4 cups corn
- ½ cup parsley, chopped
- 2 spring onions, chopped

Directions:
1. In a salad bowl, combine the corn with the onions and the rest of the ingredients, toss and serve cold.
Nutrition: calories 121, fat 9.5, fiber 1.8, carbs 4.1, protein 1.9

Radish and Corn Salad
Preparation time: 10 minutes
Cooking time: 0 minutes
Servings: 2
Ingredients:
- 1 tablespoon lemon juice
- 1 jalapeno, chopped
- 2 tablespoons olive oil
- ¼ teaspoon oregano, dried
- A pinch of sea salt and black pepper
- 2 cups fresh corn
- 6 radishes, sliced

Directions:
1. In a salad bowl, combine the corn with the radishes and the rest of the ingredients, toss and serve cold.
Nutrition: calories 134, fat 4.5, fiber 1.8, carbs 4.1, protein 1.9

Arugula and Corn Salad
Preparation time: 10 minutes
Cooking time: 0 minutes
Servings: 4
Ingredients:
- 1 red bell pepper, thinly sliced
- 2 cups corn
- Juice of 1 lime

- Zest of 1 lime, grated
- 8 cups baby arugula
- A pinch of sea salt and black pepper

Directions:
1. In a salad bowl, mix the corn with the arugula and the rest of the ingredients, toss and serve cold.
Nutrition: calories 172, fat 8.5, fiber 1.8, carbs 5.1, protein 1.4

Balsamic Bulgur Salad
Preparation time: 30 minutes
Cooking time: 0 minutes
Servings: 4
Ingredients:
- 1 cup bulgur
- 2 cups hot water
- 1 cucumber, sliced
- A pinch of sea salt and black pepper
- 2 tablespoons lemon juice
- 2 tablespoons balsamic vinegar
- ¼ cup olive oil

Directions:
1. In a bowl, mix bulgur with the water, cover, leave aside for 30 minutes, fluff with a fork and transfer to a salad bowl.
2. Add the rest of the ingredients, toss and serve.
Nutrition: calories 171, fat 5.1, fiber 6.1, carbs 11.3, protein 4.4

Lettuce and Cucumber Salad
Preparation time: 10 minutes
Cooking time: 0 minutes
Servings: 4
Ingredients:
- 2 tablespoons olive oil
- 2 cucumbers, sliced
- 1 romaine lettuce head, torn
- 1 medium tomato, chopped
- ½ teaspoon sumac
- 1 cup parsley, chopped
- Juice of 1 lime

Directions:
1. In a bowl, mix the cucumbers with the lettuce and the rest of the ingredients, toss and serve.
Nutrition: calories 133, fat 5.1, fiber 1.1, carbs 1.3, protein 4.4

Dill Cucumber and Tomato Salad
Preparation time: 20 minutes
Cooking time: 0 minutes
Servings: 6
Ingredients:
- 1 pound tomatoes, cubed
- 1 pound cucumbers, chopped
- 1 red onion, sliced
- 2 tablespoons dill, chopped
- Salt and black pepper to the taste
- 3 tablespoons olive oil
- 3 tablespoons lemon juice

Directions:

1.   In a large salad bowl mix the tomatoes with the cucumbers and the rest of the ingredients, toss and serve after keeping in the fridge for 20 minutes.
Nutrition: calories 70, fat 1.8, fiber 1.1, carbs 4.4, protein 6.6

Corn, Carrot and Rice Salad
Preparation time: 10 minutes
Cooking time: 0 minutes
Servings: 4
Ingredients:
- ½ cup brown rice, cooked
- 2 tablespoons olive oil
- 1 red onion, sliced
- 2 carrots, grated
- ½ cup mint, chopped
- Juice of 1 lime
- ½ cup corn
- Salt and black pepper to the taste
Directions:
1.   In a salad bowl, combine the rice with the onion and the rest of the ingredients, toss and serve cold.
Nutrition: calories 145, fat 5.8, fiber 6.1, carbs 9.4, protein 6.6

Peas and Couscous Salad
Preparation time: 10 minutes
Cooking time: 0 minutes
Servings: 6
Ingredients:
- 2 cups couscous, cooked
- 3 tablespoons olive oil
- 1 cup sweet peas
- ¼ cup parsley, chopped
- 1 tablespoon mint, chopped
- Salt and black pepper to the taste
Directions:
1.   In a salad bowl, combine the couscous with the peas, and the other ingredients, toss and serve.
Nutrition: calories 210, fat 2, fiber 2, carbs 4, protein 7

Yogurt Cucumber Salad
Preparation time: 1 hour
Cooking time: 0 minutes
Servings: 4
Ingredients:
- 2 garlic cloves, minced
- Salt and white pepper to the taste
- 1 tablespoon wine vinegar
- 1 cup Greek yogurt
- 1 tablespoon dill, chopped
- 3 medium cucumbers, sliced
- 1 tablespoon avocado oil
- 1 tablespoon chives, chopped
Directions:
1.   In a bowl, mix the cucumbers with the garlic, salt, pepper and the rest of the ingredients, toss and keep in the fridge for 1 hour before serving.

Nutrition: calories 210, fat 11.3, fiber 6.4, carbs 7.5, protein 3.4

Greek Potato and Corn Salad
Preparation time: 10 minutes
Cooking time: 20 minutes
Servings: 2
Ingredients:
- 2 medium potatoes, peeled and cubed
- 2 shallots, chopped
- 1 tablespoon olive oil
- 2 cups corn
- 1 tablespoon dill, chopped
- 1 tablespoon balsamic vinegar
- Salt and black pepper to the taste
Directions:
5.   Put the potatoes in a pot, add water to cover, bring to a simmer over medium heat, cook for 20 minutes, drain and transfer to a bowl.
6.   Add the shallots and the other ingredients, toss and serve cold.
Nutrition: calories 198, fat 5.3, fiber 6.5, carbs 11.6, protein 4.5

Parsley Tomato Mix
Preparation time: 10 minutes
Cooking time: 10 minutes
Servings: 4
Ingredients:
- 4 medium tomatoes, roughly cubed
- 1 garlic clove, minced
- 1 tablespoon olive oil
- ½ teaspoon sweet paprika
- Salt and black pepper to the taste
- ½ bunch parsley, chopped
Directions:
1.   Heat up a pot with the olive oil over medium heat, add the tomatoes and the garlic and sauté for 5 minutes.
2.   Add the rest of the ingredients, toss, cook for 3-4 minutes more, divide into bowls and serve.
Nutrition: calories 220, fat 9.4, fiber 5.3, carbs 6.5, protein 4.6

Garlic Cucumber Mix
Preparation time: 15 minutes
Cooking time: 0 minutes
Servings: 4
Ingredients:
- 2 cucumbers, sliced
- 2 spring onions, chopped
- 2 tablespoons olive oil
- 3 garlic cloves, grated
- 1 tablespoon thyme, chopped
- Salt and black pepper to the taste
- 3 and ½ ounces goat cheese, crumbled
Directions:
1.   In a salad bowl, mix the cucumbers with the onions and the rest of the ingredients, toss and serve after keeping it in the fridge for 15 minutes.

Nutrition: calories 140, fat 5.4, fiber 4.3, carbs 6.5, protein 4.8

Jalapeno Tomato salad

Preparation time: 10 minutes
Cooking time: 0 minutes
Servings: 4
Ingredients:
- 6 big tomatoes, peeled and cut into wedges
- 2 tablespoons olive oil
- 1 yellow onion, chopped
- 2 jalapenos, chopped
- 1 green bell pepper, chopped
- 2 garlic cloves, minced
- Salt and black pepper to the taste
- A splash of balsamic vinegar
- 1 tablespoon basil, chopped

Directions:
1. In a salad bowl, combine the tomatoes with the jalapeno, onion and the rest of the ingredients, toss and serve right away.
Nutrition: calories 200, fat 5.6, fiber 3.4, carbs 11.5, protein 6.5

Broccoli and Mushroom Salad

Preparation time: 10 minutes
Cooking time: 0 minutes
Servings: 4
Ingredients:
- ½ pound white mushrooms, sliced
- 1 broccoli head, florets separated and steamed
- 1 garlic clove, minced
- 1 tablespoon balsamic vinegar
- 1 yellow onion, chopped
- 1 tablespoon olive oil
- A pinch of sea salt and black pepper
- A pinch of red pepper flakes

Directions:
1. In a bowl, mix the broccoli with the mushrooms and the other ingredients, toss and serve cold.
Nutrition: calories 183, fat 6.5, fiber 4.2, carbs 8.5, protein 4

Avocado and Mushroom Mix

Preparation time: 10 minutes
Cooking time: 10 minutes
Servings: 4
Ingredients:
- 1 yellow onion, chopped
- 1 tablespoon balsamic vinegar
- 2 tablespoons olive oil
- 12 ounces mushrooms, sliced
- 2 avocados, pitted, peeled and cubed
- 1 garlic clove, minced
- A pinch of salt and black pepper

Directions:
1. Heat up a pan with half of the oil over medium-high heat, add the mushrooms, sauté for 10 minutes and transfer to a bowl.
2. Add the rest of the ingredients, toss and serve.

Nutrition: calories 187, fat 4.3, fiber 4.2, carbs 11.6, protein 4

Saffron Zucchini Mix

Preparation time: 10 minutes
Cooking time: 10 minutes
Servings: 4
Ingredients:
- 2 zucchinis, sliced
- A pinch of sea salt and black pepper
- 1 tablespoon white vinegar
- 1 tablespoon olive oil
- 1 teaspoon saffron powder

Directions:
1. Heat up a pan with the oil over medium heat, add the zucchinis and sauté for 8 minutes.
2. Add the rest of the ingredients, toss, cook for 2 minutes more, divide between plates and serve.
Nutrition: calories 150, fat 5.2, fiber 4.3, carbs 5, protein 4

Hemp and Cucumber Salad

Preparation time: 10 minutes
Cooking time: 0 minutes
Servings: 2
Ingredients:
- 2 cucumbers, roughly cubed
- 2 green onions, chopped
- 1 tablespoon dill, chopped
- 1 tablespoon lemon juice
- A pinch of sea salt and black pepper
- ½ cup hemp seeds
- A drizzle of olive oil

Directions:
1. In a salad bowl, combine the cucumbers with the onions and the rest of the ingredients, toss and serve cold.
Nutrition: calories 153, fat 4, fiber 5, carbs 6, protein 3.4

Minty Cauliflower Mix

Preparation time: 10 minutes
Cooking time: 0 minutes
Servings: 2
Ingredients:
- ½ cups walnuts, chopped
- 2 cups cauliflower florets, steamed
- 1 teaspoon ginger, grated
- 1 garlic clove, minced
- 1 tablespoon mint, chopped
- Juice of ½ lemon
- A pinch of sea salt and black pepper

Directions:
1. In a salad bowl, combine the cauliflower with the walnuts and the rest of the ingredients, toss and serve.
Nutrition: calories 199, fat 5.6, fiber 4.5, carbs 8.4, protein 3.5

Leeks Salad

Preparation time: 10 minutes
Cooking time: 0 minutes
Servings: 4
Ingredients:
- 1 tablespoon olive oil
- 4 leeks, sliced
- 3 garlic cloves, grated
- A pinch of sea salt and white pepper
- ½ teaspoon apple cider vinegar
- A drizzle of olive oil
- 1 tablespoon dill, chopped

Directions:
1. In a salad bowl, combine the leeks with the garlic and the rest of the ingredients, toss and serve cold.

Nutrition: calories 71, fat 2.1, fiber 1.1, carbs 1.3, protein 2.4

Snow Peas Salad

Preparation time: 6 hours
Cooking time: 10 minutes
Servings: 4
Ingredients:
- 3 cups snow peas, trimmed
- 1 and ¼ cup bean sprouts
- 1 tablespoon basil, chopped
- 1 tablespoon lime juice
- 1 teaspoon ginger, grated
- 2 spring onions, chopped
- 2 garlic cloves, minced

Directions:
1. Put the snow peas in a pot, add water to cover, bring to a simmer and cook over medium heat for 10 minutes.
2. Drain the peas, transfer them to a bowl, add the sprouts and the rest of the ingredients, toss and keep in the fridge for 6 hours before serving.

Nutrition: calories 200, fat 8.6, fiber 3, carbs 5.4, protein 3.4

Parsley Couscous and Cherries Salad

Preparation time: 10 minutes
Cooking time: 0 minutes
Servings: 6
Ingredients:
- 2 cups hot water
- 1 cup couscous
- ½ cup walnuts, roasted and chopped
- ½ cup cherries, pitted
- ½ cup parsley, chopped
- A pinch of sea salt and black pepper
- 1 tablespoon lime juice
- 2 tablespoons olive oil

Directions:
1. Put the couscous in a bowl, add the hot water, cover, leave aside for 10 minutes, fluff with a fork and transfer to a bowl.
2. Add the rest of the ingredients, toss and serve.

Nutrition: calories 200, fat 6.71, fiber 7.3, carbs 8.5, protein 5

Mango and Cucumber Salad

Preparation time: 10 minutes
Cooking time: 0 minutes
Servings: 4
Ingredients:
- 1 avocado, pitted, peeled and chopped
- ½ pound cucumbers, sliced
- 2 mangos, peeled and cubed
- 1 tablespoon olive oil
- 1 garlic clove, minced
- 2 tablespoons lime juice
- 1 teaspoon mustard
- A pinch of salt and black pepper

Directions:
1. In a salad bowl, combine the cucumbers with the mangos and the rest of the ingredients, toss and serve.

Nutrition: calories 190, fat 6, fiber 2, carbs 6.6, protein 8

Fennel and Zucchini Mix

Preparation time: 10 minutes
Cooking time: 15 minutes
Servings: 4
Ingredients:
- 1 cup fennel bulb, chopped
- 1 sweet onion, chopped
- 1 tablespoon olive oil
- 3 garlic cloves, minced
- 5 cups zucchini, roughly cubed
- 1 cup veggie stock
- Salt and black pepper the taste
- 2 teaspoons white wine vinegar
- 1 teaspoon lemon juice

Directions:
1. Heat up a pan with the oil over medium heat, add the onion and the garlic, toss and sauté for 5 minutes.
2. Add the rest of the ingredients, toss, cook for 10 minutes more, divide into bowls and serve.

Nutrition: calories 193, fat 3, fiber 2.4, carbs 3, protein 2.3

Bell Peppers Salad

Preparation time: 10 minutes
Cooking time: 0 minutes
Servings: 6
Ingredients:
- 2 green bell peppers, cut into thick strips
- 2 red bell peppers, cut into thick strips
- 2 tablespoons olive oil
- 1 garlic clove, minced
- ½ cup goat cheese, crumbled
- A pinch of salt and black pepper

Directions:
1. In a bowl, mix the bell peppers with the garlic and the other ingredients, toss and serve.

Nutrition: calories 193, fat 4.5, fiber 2, carbs 4.3, protein 3

Zucchini and Corn

Preparation time: 10 minutes
Cooking time: 15 minutes
Servings: 4
Ingredients:
- Salt and black pepper to the taste
- 2 tablespoons olive oil
- 2 zucchinis, quartered and cubed
- 1 yellow onion, chopped
- 1 cup corn kernels
- 3 tablespoons mint, chopped
- 2 teaspoons balsamic vinegar

Directions:
1. Heat up a pan with the oil over medium-high heat, add the zucchinis and sauté for 5 minutes.
2. Add the rest of the ingredients, toss, cook for 10 minutes more, divide into bowls and serve.
Nutrition: calories 120, fat 1.8, fiber 1.1, carbs 1.4, protein 2.6

Lime Beans Salad

Preparation time: 1 hour
Cooking time: 0 minutes
Servings: 4
Ingredients:
- 10 ounces canned cannellini beans, drained and rinsed
- 15 ounces canned kidney beans, drained
- Salt and black pepper to the taste
- 1 garlic clove, minced
- 10 ounces corn
- ½ cup olive oil
- 1 red onion, chopped
- 2 tablespoons lime juice
- ½ tablespoon cumin, ground
- ¼ cup cilantro, chopped

Directions:
1. In a bowl, mix the beans with salt, pepper, the garlic and the rest of the ingredients, toss and serve.
Nutrition: calories 190, fat 11.8, fiber 4.1, carbs 5.4, protein 6.6

Lettuce and Onions Salad

Preparation time: 10 minutes
Cooking time: 0 minutes
Servings: 4
Ingredients:
- ¼ cup lime juice
- 1 garlic clove, minced
- Salt and black pepper to the taste
- 2 tablespoons olive oil
- 1 green head lettuce, chopped
- 2 red onions, chopped
- 4 tomatoes, chopped
- ½ cup cilantro, chopped

Directions:

1. In a bowl, mix the lettuce with the onions and the rest of the ingredients, toss and serve right away.
Nutrition: calories 103, fat 3, fiber 2, carbs 3, protein 2

Sweet Potato and Eggplant Mix

Preparation time: 10 minutes
Cooking time: 15 minutes
Servings: 4
Ingredients:
- 2 baby eggplants, cubed
- 2 sweet potatoes, cubed
- 1 tablespoon olive oil
- 1 red onion, cut into wedges
- 1 teaspoon hot paprika
- 2 teaspoons cumin, ground
- Salt and black pepper to the taste
- 4 cups baby spinach
- ¼ cup lime juice

Directions:
1. Heat up a pan with the oil over medium-high heat, add the eggplants and the potatoes and sauté for 5 minutes.
2. Add the rest of the ingredients except the spinach, toss and cook for 10 minutes more.
3. Add the spinach, toss, divide into bowls and serve.
Nutrition: calories 200, fat 8.3, fiber 3.4, carbs 12.4, protein 4.5

Tomato and Beans Salad

Preparation time: 10 minutes
Cooking time: 0 minutes
Servings: 4
Ingredients:
- 2 tomatoes, cubed
- 2 cups canned black beans, drained and rinsed
- 1 garlic clove, minced
- 1 yellow onion, chopped
- 1 tablespoon olive oil
- Salt and black pepper to the taste
- ¼ teaspoon cumin, ground

Directions:
1. In a bowl, combine the tomatoes with the beans and the other ingredients, toss and serve.
Nutrition: calories 200, fat 8.7, fiber 3.4, carbs 6.5, protein 5.4

Cheese Avocado Salad

Preparation time: 10 minutes
Cooking time: 0 minutes
Servings: 4
Ingredients:
- Salt and black pepper to the taste
- 1 tablespoon olive oil
- 2 avocadoes, pitted, peeled and cubed
- ½ teaspoon lime juice
- 2 ounces feta cheese, crumbled
- 2 scallions, chopped
- 1 tablespoon mint, chopped

Directions:
1. In a salad bowl, combine the avocados with the scallions and the rest of the ingredients, toss and serve right away.
Nutrition: calories 222, fat 2.4, fiber 3.4, carbs 12.4, protein 4.5

Mozzarella and Pears Salad

Preparation time: 10 minutes
Cooking time: 0 minutes
Servings: 4
Ingredients:
- 1 and ½ teaspoons orange zest, grated
- ¼ cup orange juice
- 3 tablespoons balsamic vinegar
- 2 tablespoons olive oil
- Salt and black pepper to the taste
- 1 romaine lettuce head, torn
- 2 pears, cored and cut into medium wedges
- 4 ounces mozzarella, shredded

Directions:
1. In a salad bowl, combine the lettuce with the pears and the other ingredients, toss and serve cold.
Nutrition: calories 200, fat 4.5, fiber 4.2, carbs 10.4, protein 3.4

Lemony Arugula Salad

Preparation time: 10 minutes
Cooking time: 0 minutes
Servings: 4
Ingredients:
- 1 tablespoon capers, drained and chopped
- 1 and ½ tablespoons balsamic vinegar
- 1 teaspoon lemon zest, grated
- 1 tablespoon lemon juice
- 1 tablespoon olive oil
- 1 teaspoon parsley, chopped
- Salt and black pepper to the taste
- 4 cups baby arugula

Directions:
1. In a salad bowl, combine the arugula with the capers and the rest of the ingredients, toss and serve.
Nutrition: calories 143, fat 3, fiber 1.2, carbs 3.4, protein 4.5

Raisins, Endives and Herbs Salad

Preparation time: 10 minutes
Cooking time: 0 minutes
Servings: 4
Ingredients:
- 2 tablespoons olive oil
- 1 cup raisins
- 2 tablespoons lemon juice
- ¼ cup chives, chopped
- ¾ cup parsley, chopped
- ¼ cup cilantro, chopped
- Salt and black pepper to the taste
- 1 cup endives, shredded
- ¼ cup dill, chopped
- ¼ cup mint leaves, torn

- 1 tablespoon sesame seeds, toasted

Directions:
1. In a salad bowl, combine the raisins with the lemon juice, oil, chives and the rest of the ingredients, toss and serve cold.
Nutrition: calories 63, fat 2.7, fiber 0.4, carbs 2.8, protein 0.7

Radish Salad

Preparation time: 10 minutes
Cooking time: 0 minutes
Servings: 4
Ingredients:
- 1 tablespoons lemon zest, grated
- Salt and black pepper to the taste
- 2 tablespoons parsley, chopped
- A drizzle of olive oil
- 1 pound red radishes, roughly cubed
- 1 small red onion, thinly sliced
- 1/3 cup black olives, pitted and halved
- Salt and black pepper to the taste
- 1 teaspoon oregano, chopped

Directions:
1. In a salad bowl, combine the radishes with the onion, olives and the rest of the ingredients, toss and serve cold.
Nutrition: calories 68, fat 4.2, fiber 2.3, carbs 3.4, protein 2.4

Capers and Spinach Salad

Preparation time: 10 minutes
Cooking time: 0 minutes
Servings: 4
Ingredients:
- 3 garlic cloves, minced
- 2 and ½ tablespoons olive oil
- 2 teaspoons balsamic vinegar
- 1 tablespoons oregano, chopped
- Salt and black pepper to the taste
- 2 tablespoons parsley, chopped
- 1 tablespoon capers, chopped
- 1 teaspoon thyme, chopped
- ¼ teaspoon red chili flakes
- 4 cups baby spinach

Directions:
1. In a bowl, mix the spinach with the capers, garlic and the other ingredients, toss and serve cold.
Nutrition: calories 92, fat 3.4, fiber 2.3, carbs 2.9, protein 2.3

Orange Potato Salad

Preparation time: 10 minutes
Cooking time: 40 minutes
Servings: 4
Ingredients:
- 4 sweet potatoes
- 3 tablespoons olive oil
- 1/3 cup orange juice
- ½ teaspoon sumac, ground
- 1 tablespoon red wine vinegar

- Salt and black pepper to the taste
- 1 tablespoon orange zest, grated
- 2 tablespoons mint, chopped
- 1/3 cup walnuts, chopped
- 1/3 cup pomegranate seeds

Directions:
1. Put the potatoes on a lined baking sheet, introduce them in the oven at 350 degrees F, bake for 40 minutes, cool them down, peel, cut into wedges and transfer to a bowl.
2. Add the rest of the ingredients, toss, and serve cold.

Nutrition: calories 138, fat 3.5, fiber 6.2, carbs 10.4, protein 6.5

Spinach and Avocado Salad

Preparation time: 5 minutes
Cooking time: 0 minutes
Servings: 4
Ingredients:
- 2 tablespoons olive oil
- 3 tablespoons balsamic vinegar
- 1 teaspoon basil, dried
- 3 avocados, peeled, pitted and cubed
- 2 cups baby spinach
- Salt and black pepper to the taste
- 1 small red onion, chopped
- 1 tablespoon dill, chopped

Directions:
1. In a bowl, mix the avocados with the spinach, basil, and the rest of the ingredients, toss and serve right away.

Nutrition: calories 53, fat 0.3, fiber 0.5, carbs 11, protein 1

Mint Cabbage Salad

Preparation time: 10 minutes
Cooking time: 0 minutes
Servings: 4
Ingredients:
- 1 small red onion, chopped
- 1 tablespoon olive oil
- 2 tablespoons lemon juice
- 1 tablespoon lemon zest, grated
- Salt and black pepper to the taste
- 1 green cabbage head, shredded
- ½ cup mint, chopped
- ¼ cup pistachios, chopped

Directions:
1. In a salad bowl, combine the cabbage with the mint, pistachios and the rest of the ingredients, toss and serve cold.

Nutrition: calories 101, fat 4.1, fiber 3.1, carbs 4.5, protein 4.6

Carrot Salad

Preparation time: 5 minutes
Cooking time: 0 minutes

Servings: 4
Ingredients:
Juice of 1 lime
2 tablespoons olive oil
1 teaspoon ginger, grated
1 tablespoon balsamic vinegar
8 carrots, peeled and roughly grated
Salt and black pepper to the taste
½ cup almonds, toasted and sliced
½ cup mint, chopped
1 tablespoon sumac, ground

Directions:
1. In a bowl, mix the carrots with the almonds, mint, sumac and the rest of the ingredients, toss and serve cold.

Nutrition: calories 100, fat 4, fiber 4, carbs 1, protein 4

Dessert Recipes

Banana Shake Bowls

Preparation time: 5 minutes
Cooking time: 0 minutes
Servings: 4
Ingredients:
- 4 medium bananas, peeled
- 1 avocado, peeled, pitted and mashed
- ¾ cup almond milk
- ½ teaspoon vanilla extract

Directions:
1. In a blender, combine the bananas with the avocado and the other ingredients, pulse, divide into bowls and keep in the fridge until serving.
Nutrition: calories 185, fat 4.3, fiber 4, carbs 6, protein 6.45

Cold Lemon Squares

Preparation time: 30 minutes
Cooking time: 0 minutes
Servings: 4
Ingredients:
- 1 cup avocado oil+ a drizzle
- 2 bananas, peeled and chopped
- 1 tablespoon honey
- ¼ cup lemon juice
- A pinch of lemon zest, grated

Directions:
1. In your food processor, mix the bananas with the rest of the ingredients, pulse well and spread on the bottom of a pan greased with a drizzle of oil.
2. Introduce in the fridge for 30 minutes, slice into squares and serve.
Nutrition: calories 136, fat 11.2, fiber 0.2, carbs 7, protein 1.1

Blackberry and Apples Cobbler

Preparation time: 10 minutes
Cooking time: 30 minutes
Servings: 6
Ingredients:
- ¾ cup stevia
- 6 cups blackberries
- ¼ cup apples, cored and cubed
- ¼ teaspoon baking powder
- 1 tablespoon lime juice
- ½ cup almond flour
- ½ cup water
- 3 and ½ tablespoon avocado oil
- Cooking spray

Directions:
1. In a bowl, mix the berries with half of the stevia and lemon juice, sprinkle some flour all over, whisk and pour into a baking dish greased with cooking spray.
2. In another bowl, mix flour with the rest of the sugar, baking powder, the water and the oil, and stir the whole thing with your hands.

3. Spread over the berries, introduce in the oven at 375 degrees F and bake for 30 minutes.
4. Serve warm.
Nutrition: calories 221, fat 6.3, fiber 3.3, carbs 6, protein 9

Black Tea Cake

Preparation time: 10 minutes
Cooking time: 35 minutes
Servings: 8
Ingredients:
- 6 tablespoons black tea powder
- 2 cups almond milk, warmed up
- 1 cup avocado oil
- 2 cups stevia
- 4 eggs
- 2 teaspoons vanilla extract
- 3 and ½ cups almond flour
- 1 teaspoon baking soda
- 3 teaspoons baking powder

Directions:
1. In a bowl, combine the almond milk with the oil, stevia and the rest of the ingredients and whisk well.
2. Pour this into a cake pan lined with parchment paper, introduce in the oven at 350 degrees F and bake for 35 minutes.
3. Leave the cake to cool down, slice and serve.
Nutrition: calories 200, fat 6.4, fiber 4, carbs 6.5, protein 5.4

Green Tea and Vanilla Cream

Preparation time: 2 hours
Cooking time: 0 minutes
Servings: 4
Ingredients:
- 14 ounces almond milk, hot
- 2 tablespoons green tea powder
- 14 ounces heavy cream
- 3 tablespoons stevia
- 1 teaspoon vanilla extract
- 1 teaspoon gelatin powder

Directions:
1. In a bowl, combine the almond milk with the green tea powder and the rest of the ingredients, whisk well, cool down, divide into cups and keep in the fridge for 2 hours before serving.
Nutrition: calories 120, fat 3, fiber 3, carbs 7, protein 4

Figs Pie

Preparation time: 10 minutes
Cooking time: 1 hour
Servings: 8
Ingredients:
- ½ cup stevia
- 6 figs, cut into quarters
- ½ teaspoon vanilla extract
- 1 cup almond flour
- 4 eggs, whisked

Directions:

1.   Spread the figs on the bottom of a springform pan lined with parchment paper.
2.   In a bowl, combine the other ingredients, whisk and pour over the figs,
3.   Bake at 375 digress F for 1 hour, flip the pie upside down when it's done and serve.
Nutrition: calories 200, fat 4.4, fiber 3, carbs 7.6, protein 8

Cherry Cream

Preparation time: 2 hours
Cooking time: 0 minutes
Servings: 4
Ingredients:
- 2 cups cherries, pitted and chopped
- 1 cup almond milk
- ½ cup whipping cream
- 3 eggs, whisked
- 1/3 cup stevia
- 1 teaspoon lemon juice
- ½ teaspoon vanilla extract

Directions:
1.   In your food processor, combine the cherries with the milk and the rest of the ingredients, pulse well, divide into cups and keep in the fridge for 2 hours before serving.
Nutrition: calories 200, fat 4.5, fiber 3.3, carbs 5.6, protein 3.4

Strawberries Cream

Preparation time: 10 minutes
Cooking time: 20 minutes
Servings: 4
Ingredients:
- ½ cup stevia
- 2 pounds strawberries, chopped
- 1 cup almond milk
- Zest of 1 lemon, grated
- ½ cup heavy cream
- 3 egg yolks, whisked

Directions:
1.   Heat up a pan with the milk over medium-high heat, add the stevia and the rest of the ingredients, whisk well, simmer for 20 minutes, divide into cups and serve cold.
Nutrition: calories 152, fat 4.4, fiber 5.5, carbs 5.1, protein 0.8

Apples and Plum Cake

Preparation time: 10 minutes
Cooking time: 40 minutes
Servings: 4
Ingredients:
- 7 ounces almond flour
- 1 egg, whisked
- 5 tablespoons stevia
- 3 ounces warm almond milk
- 2 pounds plums, pitted and cut into quarters
- 2 apples, cored and chopped
- Zest of 1 lemon, grated

- 1 teaspoon baking powder
Directions:
1.   In a bowl, mix the almond milk with the egg, stevia, and the rest of the ingredients except the cooking spray and whisk well.
2.   Grease a cake pan with the oil, pour the cake mix inside, introduce in the oven and bake at 350 degrees F for 40 minutes.
3.   Cool down, slice and serve.
Nutrition: calories 209, fat 6.4, fiber 6, carbs 8, protein 6.6

Cinnamon Chickpeas Cookies

Preparation time: 10 minutes
Cooking time: 20 minutes
Servings: 12
Ingredients:
- 1 cup canned chickpeas, drained, rinsed and mashed
- 2 cups almond flour
- 1 teaspoon cinnamon powder
- 1 teaspoon baking powder
- 1 cup avocado oil
- ½ cup stevia
- 1 egg, whisked
- 2 teaspoons almond extract
- 1 cup raisins
- 1 cup coconut, unsweetened and shredded

Directions:
1.   In a bowl, combine the chickpeas with the flour, cinnamon and the other ingredients, and whisk well until you obtain a dough.
2.   Scoop tablespoons of dough on a baking sheet lined with parchment paper, introduce them in the oven at 350 degrees F and bake for 20 minutes.
3.   Leave them to cool down for a few minutes and serve.
Nutrition: calories 200, fat 4.5, fiber 3.4, carbs 9.5, protein 2.4

Cocoa Brownies

Preparation time: 10 minutes
Cooking time: 20 minutes
Servings: 8
Ingredients:
- 30 ounces canned lentils, rinsed and drained
- 1 tablespoon honey
- 1 banana, peeled and chopped
- ½ teaspoon baking soda
- 4 tablespoons almond butter
- 2 tablespoons cocoa powder
- Cooking spray

Directions:
1.   In a food processor, combine the lentils with the honey and the other ingredients except the cooking spray and pulse well.
2.   Pour this into a pan greased with cooking spray, spread evenly, introduce in the oven at 375 degrees F and bake for 20 minutes.
3.   Cut the brownies and serve cold.

Nutrition: calories 200, fat 4.5, fiber 2.4 carbs 8.7, protein 4.3

Cardamom Almond Cream

Preparation time: 30 minutes
Cooking time: 0 minutes
Servings: 4
Ingredients:
- Juice of 1 lime
- ½ cup stevia
- 1 and ½ cups water
- 3 cups almond milk
- ½ cup honey
- 2 teaspoons cardamom, ground
- 1 teaspoon rose water
- 1 teaspoon vanilla extract

Directions:
1. In a blender, combine the almond milk with the cardamom and the rest of the ingredients, pulse well, divide into cups and keep in the fridge for 30 minutes before serving.
Nutrition: calories 283, fat 11.8, fiber 0.3, carbs 4.7, protein 7.1

Banana Cinnamon Cupcakes

Preparation time: 10 minutes
Cooking time: 20 minutes
Servings: 4
Ingredients:
- 4 tablespoons avocado oil
- 4 eggs
- ½ cup orange juice
- 2 teaspoons cinnamon powder
- 1 teaspoon vanilla extract
- 2 bananas, peeled and chopped
- ¾ cup almond flour
- ½ teaspoon baking powder
- Cooking spray

Directions:
1. In a bowl, combine the oil with the eggs, orange juice and the other ingredients except the cooking spray, whisk well, pour in a cupcake pan greased with the cooking spray, introduce in the oven at 350 degrees F and bake for 20 minutes.
2. Cool the cupcakes down and serve.
Nutrition: calories 142, fat 5.8, fiber 4.2, carbs 5.7, protein 1.6

Rhubarb and Apples Cream

Preparation time: 10 minutes
Cooking time: 0 minutes
Servings: 6
Ingredients:
- 3 cups rhubarb, chopped
- 1 and ½ cups stevia
- 2 eggs, whisked
- ½ teaspoon nutmeg, ground
- 1 tablespoon avocado oil
- 1/3 cup almond milk

Directions:

1. In a blender, combine the rhubarb with the stevia and the rest of the ingredients, pulse well, divide into cups and serve cold.
Nutrition: calories 200, fat 5.2, fiber 3.4, carbs 7.6, protein 2.5

Almond Rice Dessert

Preparation time: 10 minutes
Cooking time: 20 minutes
Servings: 4
Ingredients:
- 1 cup white rice
- 2 cups almond milk
- 1 cup almonds, chopped
- ½ cup stevia
- 1 tablespoon cinnamon powder
- ½ cup pomegranate seeds

Directions:
1. In a pot, mix the rice with the milk and stevia, bring to a simmer and cook for 20 minutes, stirring often.
2. Add the rest of the ingredients, stir, divide into bowls and serve.
Nutrition: calories 234, fat 9.5, fiber 3.4, carbs 12.4, protein 6.5

Peach Sorbet

Preparation time: 2 hours
Cooking time: 10 minutes
Servings: 4
Ingredients:
- 2 cups apple juice
- 1 cup stevia
- 2 tablespoons lemon zest, grated
- 2 pounds peaches, pitted and quartered

Directions:
1. Heat up a pan over medium heat, add the apple juice and the rest of the ingredients, simmer for 10 minutes, transfer to a blender, pulse, divide into cups and keep in the freezer for 2 hours before serving.
Nutrition: calories 182, fat 5.4, fiber 3.4, carbs 12, protein 5.4

Cranberries and Pears Pie

Preparation time: 10 minutes
Cooking time: 40 minutes
Servings: 4
Ingredients:
- 2 cup cranberries
- 3 cups pears, cubed
- A drizzle of olive oil
- 1 cup stevia
- 1/3 cup almond flour
- 1 cup rolled oats
- ¼ avocado oil

Directions:
1. In a bowl, mix the cranberries with the pears and the other ingredients except the olive oil and the oats, and stir well.

2. Grease a cake pan with the a drizzle of olive oil, pour the pears mix inside, sprinkle the oats all over and bake at 350 degrees F for 40 minutes.
3. Cool the mix down, and serve.
Nutrition: calories 172, fat 3.4, fiber 4.3, carbs 11.5, protein 4.5

Lemon Cream

Preparation time: 1 hour
Cooking time: 10 minutes
Servings: 6
Ingredients:
- 2 eggs, whisked
- 1 and ¼ cup stevia
- 10 tablespoons avocado oil
- 1 cup heavy cream
- Juice of 2 lemons
- Zest of 2 lemons, grated

Directions:
1. In a pan, combine the cream with the lemon juice and the other ingredients, whisk well, cook for 10 minutes, divide into cups and keep in the fridge for 1 hour before serving.
Nutrition: calories 200, fat 8.5, fiber 4.5, carbs 8.6, protein 4.5

Blueberries Stew

Preparation time: 10 minutes
Cooking time: 10 minutes
Servings: 4
Ingredients:
- 2 cups blueberries
- 3 tablespoons stevia
- 1 and ½ cups pure apple juice
- 1 teaspoon vanilla extract

Directions:
1. In a pan, combine the blueberries with stevia and the other ingredients, bring to a simmer and cook over medium-low heat for 10 minutes.
2. Divide into cups and serve cold.
Nutrition: calories 192, fat 5.4, fiber 3.4, carbs 9.4, protein 4.5

Mandarin Cream

Preparation time: 20 minutes
Cooking time: 0 minutes
Servings: 8
Ingredients:
- 2 mandarins, peeled and cut into segments
- Juice of 2 mandarins
- 2 tablespoons stevia
- 4 eggs, whisked
- ¾ cup stevia
- ¾ cup almonds, ground

Directions:
1. In a blender, combine the mandarins with the mandarins juice and the other ingredients, whisk well, divide into cups and keep in the fridge for 20 minutes before serving.
Nutrition: calories 106, fat 3.4, fiber 0, carbs 2.4, protein 4

Creamy Mint Strawberry Mix

Preparation time: 10 minutes
Cooking time: 30 minutes
Servings: 6
Ingredients:
- Cooking spray
- ¼ cup stevia
- 1 and ½ cup almond flour
- 1 teaspoon baking powder
- 1 cup almond milk
- 1 egg, whisked
- 2 cups strawberries, sliced
- 1 tablespoon mint, chopped
- 1 teaspoon lime zest, grated
- ½ cup whipping cream

Directions:
1. In a bowl, combine the almond with the strawberries, mint and the other ingredients except the cooking spray and whisk well.
2. Grease 6 ramekins with the cooking spray, pour the strawberry mix inside, introduce in the oven and bake at 350 degrees F for 30 minutes.
3. Cool down and serve.
Nutrition: calories 200, fat 6.3, fiber 2, carbs 6.5, protein 8

Vanilla Cake

Preparation time: 10 minutes
Cooking time: 25 minutes
Servings: 10
Ingredients:
- 3 cups almond flour
- 3 teaspoons baking powder
- 1 cup olive oil
- 1 and ½ cup almond milk
- 1 and 2/3 cup stevia
- 2 cups water
- 1 tablespoon lime juice
- 2 teaspoons vanilla extract
- Cooking spray

Directions:
1. In a bowl, mix the almond flour with the baking powder, the oil and the rest of the ingredients except the cooking spray and whisk well.
2. Pour the mix into a cake pan greased with the cooking spray, introduce in the oven and bake at 370 degrees F for 25 minutes.
3. Leave the cake to cool down, cut and serve!
Nutrition: calories 200, fat 7.6, fiber 2.5, carbs 5.5, protein 4.5

Pumpkin Cream

Preparation time: 5 minutes
Cooking time: 5 minutes
Servings: 2
Ingredients:
- 2 cups canned pumpkin flesh
- 2 tablespoons stevia
- 1 teaspoon vanilla extract
- 2 tablespoons water

- A pinch of pumpkin spice

Directions:

1. In a pan, combine the pumpkin flesh with the other ingredients, simmer for 5 minutes, divide into cups and serve cold.

Nutrition: calories 192, fat 3.4, fiber 4.5, carbs 7.6, protein 3.5

Chia and Berries Smoothie Bowl

Preparation time: 5 minutes
Cooking time: 0 minutes
Servings: 2
Ingredients:

- 1 and ½ cup almond milk
- 1 cup blackberries
- ¼ cup strawberries, chopped
- 1 and ½ tablespoons chia seeds
- 1 teaspoon cinnamon powder

Directions:

1. In a blender, combine the blackberries with the strawberries and the rest of the ingredients, pulse well, divide into small bowls and serve cold.

Nutrition: calories 182, fat 3.4, fiber 3.4, carbs 8.4, protein 3

Minty Coconut Cream

Preparation time: 4 minutes
Cooking time: 0 minutes
Servings: 2
Ingredients:

- 1 banana, peeled
- 2 cups coconut flesh, shredded
- 3 tablespoons mint, chopped
- 1 and ½ cups coconut water
- 2 tablespoons stevia
- ½ avocado, pitted and peeled

Directions:

1. In a blender, combine the coconut with the banana and the rest of the ingredients, pulse well, divide into cups and serve cold.

Nutrition: calories 193, fat 5.4, fiber 3.4, carbs 7.6, protein 3

Watermelon Cream

Preparation time: 15 minutes
Cooking time: 0 minutes
Servings: 2
Ingredients:

- 1 pound watermelon, peeled and chopped
- 1 teaspoon vanilla extract
- 1 cup heavy cream
- 1 teaspoon lime juice
- 2 tablespoons stevia

Directions:

1. In a blender, combine the watermelon with the cream and the rest of the ingredients, pulse well, divide into cups and keep in the fridge for 15 minutes before serving.

Nutrition: calories 122, fat 5.7, fiber 3.2, carbs 5.3, protein 0.4

Grapes Stew

Preparation time: 10 minutes
Cooking time: 10 minutes
Servings: 4
Ingredients:

- 2/3 cup stevia
- 1 tablespoon olive oil
- 1/3 cup coconut water
- 1 teaspoon vanilla extract
- 1 teaspoon lemon zest, grated
- 2 cup red grapes, halved

Directions:

1. Heat up a pan with the water over medium heat, add the oil, stevia and the rest of the ingredients, toss, simmer for 10 minutes, divide into cups and serve.

Nutrition: calories 122, fat 3.7, fiber 1.2, carbs 2.3, protein 0.4

Cocoa Sweet Cherry Cream

Preparation time: 2 hours
Cooking time: 0 minutes
Servings: 4
Ingredients:

- ½ cup cocoa powder
- ¾ cup red cherry jam
- ¼ cup stevia
- 2 cups water
- 1 pound cherries, pitted and halved

Directions:

1. In a blender, mix the cherries with the water and the rest of the ingredients, pulse well, divide into cups and keep in the fridge for 2 hours before serving.

Nutrition: calories 162, fat 3.4, fiber 2.4, carbs 5, protein 1

Apple Couscous Pudding

Preparation time: 10 minutes
Cooking time: 25 minutes
Servings: 4
Ingredients:

- ½ cup couscous
- 1 and ½ cups milk
- ¼ cup apple, cored and chopped
- 3 tablespoons stevia
- ½ teaspoon rose water
- 1 tablespoon orange zest, grated

Directions:

1. Heat up a pan with the milk over medium heat, add the couscous and the rest of the ingredients, whisk, simmer for 25 minutes, divide into bowls and serve.

Nutrition: calories 150, fat 4.5, fiber 5.5, carbs 7.5, protein 4

Ricotta Ramekins

Preparation time: 10 minutes
Cooking time: 1 hour
Servings: 4
Ingredients:

- 6 eggs, whisked

- 1 and ½ pounds ricotta cheese, soft
- ½ pound stevia
- 1 teaspoon vanilla extract
- ½ teaspoon baking powder
- Cooking spray

Directions:

1. In a bowl, mix the eggs with the ricotta and the other ingredients except the cooking spray and whisk well.
2. Grease 4 ramekins with the cooking spray, pour the ricotta cream in each and bake at 360 degrees F for 1 hour.
3. Serve cold.

Nutrition: calories 180, fat 5.3, fiber 5.4, carbs 11.5, protein 4

Papaya Cream

Preparation time: 10 minutes
Cooking time: 0 minutes
Servings: 2
Ingredients:

- 1 cup papaya, peeled and chopped
- 1 cup heavy cream
- 1 tablespoon stevia
- ½ teaspoon vanilla extract

Directions:

1. In a blender, combine the cream with the papaya and the other ingredients, pulse well, divide into cups and serve cold.

Nutrition: calories 182, fat 3.1, fiber 2.3, carbs 3.5, protein 2

Almonds and Oats Pudding

Preparation time: 10 minutes
Cooking time: 15 minutes
Servings: 4
Ingredients:

- 1 tablespoon lemon juice
- Zest of 1 lime
- 1 and ½ cups almond milk
- 1 teaspoon almond extract
- ½ cup oats
- 2 tablespoons stevia
- ½ cup silver almonds, chopped

Directions:

1. In a pan, combine the almond milk with the lime zest and the other ingredients, whisk, bring to a simmer and cook over medium heat for 15 minutes.
2. Divide the mix into bowls and serve cold.

Nutrition: calories 174, fat 12.1, fiber 3.2, carbs 3.9, protein 4.8

Chocolate Cups

Preparation time: 2 hours
Cooking time: 0 minutes
Servings: 6
Ingredients:

- ½ cup avocado oil
- 1 cup, chocolate, melted
- 1 teaspoon matcha powder

- 3 tablespoons stevia

Directions:

1. In a bowl, mix the chocolate with the oil and the rest of the ingredients, whisk really well, divide into cups and keep in the freezer for 2 hours before serving.

Nutrition: calories 174, fat 9.1, fiber 2.2, carbs 3.9, protein 2.8

Mango Bowls

Preparation time: 30 minutes
Cooking time: 0 minutes
Servings: 4
Ingredients:

- 3 cups mango, cut into medium chunks
- ½ cup coconut water
- ¼ cup stevia
- 1 teaspoon vanilla extract

Directions:

1. In a blender, combine the mango with the rest of the ingredients, pulse well, divide into bowls and serve cold.

Nutrition: calories 122, fat 4, fiber 5.3, carbs 6.6, protein 4.5

Cocoa and Pears Cream

Preparation time: 10 minutes
Cooking time: 0 minutes
Servings: 4
Ingredients:

- 2 cups heavy creamy
- 1/3 cup stevia
- ¾ cup cocoa powder
- 6 ounces dark chocolate, chopped
- Zest of 1 lemon
- 2 pears, chopped

Directions:

1. In a blender, combine the cream with the stevia and the rest of the ingredients, pulse well, divide into cups and serve cold.

Nutrition: calories 172, fat 5.6, fiber 3.5, carbs 7.6, protein 4

Pineapple Pudding

Preparation time: 10 minutes
Cooking time: 40 minutes
Servings: 4
Ingredients:

- 3 cups almond flour
- ¼ cup olive oil
- 1 teaspoon vanilla extract
- 2 and ¼ cups stevia
- 3 eggs, whisked
- 1 and ¼ cup natural apple sauce
- 2 teaspoons baking powder
- 1 and ¼ cups almond milk
- 2 cups pineapple, chopped
- Cooking spray

Directions:

1. In a bowl, combine the almond flour with the oil and the rest of the ingredients except the cooking spray and stir well.
2. Grease a cake pan with the cooking spray, pour the pudding mix inside, introduce in the oven and bake at 370 degrees F for 40 minutes.
3. Serve the pudding cold.
Nutrition: calories 223, fat 8.1, fiber 3.4, carbs 7.6, protein 3.4

Lime Vanilla Fudge
Preparation time: 3 hours
Cooking time: 0 minutes
Servings: 6
Ingredients:
- 1/3 cup cashew butter
- 5 tablespoons lime juice
- ½ teaspoon lime zest, grated
- 1 tablespoons stevia

Directions:
1. In a bowl, mix the cashew butter with the other ingredients and whisk well.
2. Line a muffin tray with parchment paper, scoop 1 tablespoon of lime fudge mix in each of the muffin tins and keep in the freezer for 3 hours before serving.
Nutrition: calories 200, fat 4.5, fiber 3.4, carbs 13.5, protein 5

Mixed Berries Stew
Preparation time: 10 minutes
Cooking time: 15 minutes
Servings: 6
Ingredients:
- Zest of 1 lemon, grated
- Juice of 1 lemon
- ½ pint blueberries
- 1 pint strawberries, halved
- 2 cups water
- 2 tablespoons stevia

Directions:
1. In a pan, combine the berries with the water, stevia and the other ingredients, bring to a simmer, cook over medium heat for 15 minutes, divide into bowls and serve cold.
Nutrition: calories 172, fat 7, fiber 3.4, carbs 8, protein 2.3

Orange and Apricots Cake
Preparation time: 10 minutes
Cooking time: 20 minutes
Servings: 8
Ingredients:
- ¾ cup stevia
- 2 cups almond flour
- ¼ cup olive oil
- ½ cup almond milk
- 1 teaspoon baking powder
- 2 eggs
- ½ teaspoon vanilla extract
- Juice and zest of 2 oranges
- 2 cups apricots, chopped

Directions:
1. In a bowl, mix the stevia with the flour and the rest of the ingredients, whisk and pour into a cake pan lined with parchment paper.
2. Introduce in the oven at 375 degrees F, bake for 20 minutes, cool down, slice and serve.
Nutrition: calories 221, fat 8.3, fiber 3.4, carbs 14.5, protein 5

Blueberry Cake
Preparation time: 10 minutes
Cooking time: 30 minutes
Servings: 6
Ingredients:
- 2 cups almond flour
- 3 cups blueberries
- 1 cup walnuts, chopped
- 3 tablespoons stevia
- 1 teaspoon vanilla extract
- 2 eggs, whisked
- 2 tablespoons avocado oil
- 1 teaspoon baking powder
- Cooking spray

Directions:
1. In a bowl, combine the flour with the blueberries, walnuts and the other ingredients except the cooking spray, and stir well.
2. Grease a cake pan with the cooking spray, pour the cake mix inside, introduce everything in the oven at 350 degrees F and bake for 30 minutes.
3. Cool the cake down, slice and serve.
Nutrition: calories 225, fat 9, fiber 4.5, carbs 10.2, protein 4.5

Blueberry Yogurt Mousse
Preparation time: 30 minutes
Cooking time: 0 minutes
Servings: 4
Ingredients:
- 2 cups Greek yogurt
- ¼ cup stevia
- ¾ cup heavy cream
- 2 cups blueberries

Directions:
1. In a blender, combine the yogurt with the other ingredients, pulse well, divide into cups and keep in the fridge for 30 minutes before serving.
Nutrition: calories 141, fat 4.7, fiber 4.7, carbs 8.3, protein 0.8

Almond Peaches Mix
Preparation time: 10 minutes
Cooking time: 10 minutes
Servings: 4
Ingredients:
- 1/3 cup almonds, toasted
- 1/3 cup pistachios, toasted
- 1 teaspoon mint, chopped

- ½ cup coconut water
- 1 teaspoon lemon zest, grated
- 4 peaches, halved
- 2 tablespoons stevia

Directions:

1. In a pan, combine the peaches with the stevia and the rest of the ingredients, simmer over medium heat for 10 minutes, divide into bowls and serve cold.

Nutrition: calories 135, fat 4.1, fiber 3.8, carbs 4.1, protein 2.3

Walnuts Cake

Preparation time: 10 minutes
Cooking time: 40 minutes
Servings: 4
Ingredients:

- ½ pound walnuts, minced
- Zest of 1 orange, grated
- 1 and ¼ cups stevia
- eggs, whisked
- 1 teaspoon almond extract
- 1 and ½ cup almond flour
- 1 teaspoon baking soda

Directions:

1. In a bowl, combine the walnuts with the orange zest and the other ingredients, whisk well and pour into a cake pan lined with parchment paper.
2. Introduce in the oven at 350 degrees F, bake for 40 minutes, cool down, slice and serve.

Nutrition: calories 205, fat 14.1, fiber 7.8, carbs 9.1, protein 3.4

Hazelnut Pudding

Preparation time: 10 minutes
Cooking time: 40 minutes
Servings: 8
Ingredients:

- 2 and ¼ cups almond flour
- 3 tablespoons hazelnuts, chopped
- 5 eggs, whisked
- 1 cup stevia
- 1 and 1/3 cups Greek yogurt
- 1 teaspoon baking powder
- 1 teaspoon vanilla extract

Directions:

1. In a bowl, combine the flour with the hazelnuts and the other ingredients, whisk well, and pour into a cake pan lined with parchment paper,
2. Introduce in the oven at 350 degrees F, bake for 30 minutes, cool down, slice and serve.

Nutrition: calories 178, fat 8.4, fiber 8.2, carbs 11.5, protein 1.4

Cinnamon Banana and Semolina Pudding

Preparation time: 5 minutes
Cooking time: 7 minutes
Servings: 6
Ingredients:

- 2 cups semolina, ground

- 1 cup olive oil
- 4 cups hot water
- 2 bananas, peeled and chopped
- 1 teaspoon cinnamon powder
- 4 tablespoons stevia

Directions:

1. Heat up a pan with the oil over medium high heat, add the semolina and brown it for 3 minutes stirring often.
2. Add the water and the rest of the ingredients except the cinnamon, stir, and simmer for 4 minutes more.
3. Divide into bowls, sprinkle the cinnamon on top and serve.

Nutrition: calories 162, fat 8, fiber 4.2, carbs 4.3, protein 8.4

Greek Raisins and Vanilla Cream

Preparation time: 2 hours
Cooking time: 0
Servings: 4
Ingredients:

- 1 cup heavy cream
- 2 cups Greek yogurt
- 3 tablespoons stevia
- 2 tablespoons raisins
- 2 tablespoons lime juice

Directions:

1. In a blender, combine the cream with the yogurt and the rest of the ingredients, pulse well, divide into cups and keep in the fridge for 2 hours before serving.

Nutrition: calories 192, fat 6.5, fiber 3.4, carbs 9.5, protein 5

Baked Peaches

Preparation time: 10 minutes
Cooking time: 30 minutes
Servings: 4
Ingredients:

- 4 teaspoons stevia
- 4 peaches, halved and pitted
- 1 teaspoon vanilla extract
- 3 tablespoons honey

Directions:

1. Arrange the peaches on a baking sheet lined with parchment paper, add the stevia, honey and vanilla and bake at 350 degrees F for 30 minutes.
2. Divide them between plates and serve.

Nutrition: calories 176, fat 4.5, fiber 7.6, carbs 11.5, protein 5

Cocoa Yogurt Mix

Preparation time: 10 minutes
Cooking time: 0 minutes
Servings: 2
Ingredients:

- 1 tablespoon cocoa powder
- ¼ cup strawberries, chopped
- ¾ cup Greek yogurt

- 5 drops vanilla stevia

Directions:
1. In a bowl, mix the yogurt with the cocoa, strawberries and the stevia and whisk well.
2. Divide the mix into bowls and serve.

Nutrition: calories 200, fat 8, fiber 3.4, carbs 7.6, protein 4.3

Nutmeg Lemon Pudding

Preparation time: 10 minutes
Cooking time: 20 minutes
Servings: 6
Ingredients:
- 2 tablespoons lemon marmalade
- 4 eggs, whisked
- 2 tablespoons stevia
- 3 cups almond milk
- 4 allspice berries, crushed
- ¼ teaspoon nutmeg, grated

Directions:
1. In a bowl, mix the lemon marmalade with the eggs and the other ingredients and whisk well.
2. Divide the mix into ramekins, introduce in the oven and bake at 350 degrees F for 20 minutes.

3. Serve cold.
Nutrition: calories 220, fat 6.6, fiber 3.4, carbs 12.4, protein 3.4

Lime Apple Pudding

Preparation time: 10 minutes
Cooking time: 15 minutes
Servings: 4
Ingredients:
- ¾ cup stevia
- 2 and ½ cups almond milk
- 3 egg yolks, whisked
- Juice of 2 limes
- 1 cup apples, cored and cubed
- Zest of 2 limes, grated

Directions:
1. In a bowl, mix the stevia with the milk and the other ingredients and whisk well.
2. Divide into ramekins, introduce in the oven and cook at 380 degrees F for 15 minutes.
3. Serve the pudding cold.
Nutrition: calories 199, fat 5.4, fiber 3.4, carbs 11.5, protein 5.6

Appendix:Recipes Index

Chicken Skillet 28
Chicken Stuffed Peppers 29
Chicken Wings and Dates Mix 87
Chicken with Artichokes and Beans 94
Chicken Wrap 80
Chicken, Carrots and Lentils Soup 40
Chicken, Corn and Peppers 82
Chickpeas and Beets Mix 46
Chickpeas and Eggplant Bowls 64
Chickpeas and Millet Stew 28
Chickpeas Salsa 61
Chickpeas Soup 35
Chickpeas, Corn and Black Beans Salad 111
Chickpeas, Figs and Couscous 50
Chili Cabbage and Coconut 50
Chili Calamari and Veggie Mix 74
Chili Chicken Mix 81
Chili Mango and Watermelon Salsa 60
Chili Pork Meatballs 103
Chili Watermelon Soup 38
Chipotle Turkey and Tomatoes 83
Chives Chicken and Radishes 86
Chives Rice Mix 54
Chocolate Cups 125
Chorizo Shrimp and Salmon Mix 76
Cilantro Pork and Olives 108
Cinnamon and Coriander Lamb 106
Cinnamon Apple and Lentils Porridge 24
Cinnamon Banana and Semolina Pudding 127
Cinnamon Chickpeas Cookies 121
Cinnamon Duck Mix 89
Cocoa and Pears Cream 125
Cocoa Brownies 121
Cocoa Sweet Cherry Cream 124
Cocoa Yogurt Mix 127
Cod and Brussels Sprouts 78
Cod and Cabbage 73
Cod and Mushrooms Mix 70
Cold Lemon Squares 120
Coriander and Coconut Chicken 92
Coriander Falafel 58
Coriander Mushroom Salad 23
Coriander Pork and Chickpeas Stew 43
Corn and Olives 55
Corn and Shrimp Salad 19
Corn and Tomato Salad 112
Corn, Carrot and Rice Salad 114
Cottage Cheese and Berries Omelet 23
Couscous and Chickpeas Bowls 19
Cranberries and Pears Pie 122
Cranberry and Dates Squares 22
Cranberry Bulgur Mix 111
Creamy Chicken and Grapes 84
Creamy Chicken And Mushrooms 86
Creamy Chicken Soup 40
Creamy Coriander Chicken 88
Creamy Curry Salmon 71
Creamy Mint Strawberry Mix 123
Creamy Pork and Turnips Mix 101
Creamy Salmon Soup 40

Creamy Spinach and Shallots Dip 61
Creamy Sweet Potatoes Mix 46
Cucumber Bites 59
Cucumber Rolls 60
Cucumber Sandwich Bites 60
Curry Chicken, Artichokes and Olives 87

D

Dill Beets Salad 48
Dill Cucumber and Tomato Salad 113
Dill Cucumber Salad 51
Duck and Blackberries 89
Duck and Orange Warm Salad 89
Duck and Tomato Sauce 88
Duck, Cucumber and Mango Salad 90

E

Eggplant and Bell Pepper Mix 51
Eggplant And Capers Dip 65
Eggplant Bites 64
Eggplant Bombs 63
Eggplant Dip 59
Eggs with Zucchini Noodles 13
Eggs, Mint and Tomatoes 26
Endives, Fennel and Orange Salad 22

F

Farro Salad 22
Fennel and Walnuts Salad 52
Fennel and Zucchini Mix 116
Fennel Pork 100
Feta Artichoke Dip 61
Feta Chicken and Cabbage 86
Figs Pie 120
Fish and Orzo 67
Fish and Tomato Sauce 67
Fish Cakes 68
Fish Soup 34

G

Garbanzo Bean Salad 19
Garlic Chicken and Endives 86
Garlic Cucumber Mix 114
Garlic Lamb and Peppers 105
Garlic Scallops and Peas Mix 76
Garlic Snap Peas Mix 55
Ginger and Cream Cheese Dip 61
Ginger Duck Mix 90
Ginger Trout and Eggplant 79
Glazed Pork Chops 96
Goat Cheese and Chives Spread 61
Grapes Stew 124
Grapes, Cucumbers and Almonds Soup 39
Greek Beans Tortillas 25
Greek Lamb And Eggplant 107
Greek Potato and Corn Salad 114
Greek Raisins and Vanilla Cream 127
Greek Trout Spread 74
Green Beans and Peppers Mix 54
Green Tea and Vanilla Cream 120
Grilled Pork Chops and Mango Mix 98
Ground Lamb Pan 101

CPSIA information can be obtained
at www.ICGtesting.com
Printed in the USA
LVHW101600250920
667082LV00030B/372